I0704854

CONTENT

PART I: PROBIOTICS AND GENERAL HEALTH

PART II: PROBIOTICS AND ORAL HEALTH

PART I

PROBIOTICS AND GENERAL

HEALTH

INTRODUCTION

Probiotic is a phrase of the modern era, denotation "for life" and is in use to name bacterial association with beneficial effects on human and animal health[1]. The reported beneficial effects of probiotic consumption include improvement of intestinal health, amelioration of symptoms of lactose intolerance, and reduction of the risk of various other diseases. Several well-characterized strains of Lactobacilli and Bifidobacteria are available for human use [2,3]. Together they play an important role in the protection of the organism against harmful microorganisms and also strengthen the host's immune system. Probiotics can be found in dairy and non-dairy products. They are usually consumed after the antibiotic therapy (for some illnesses), which destroys the microbial flora present in the digestive tract (both the useful and the targeted harmful microbes). Regular consumption of food containing probiotic microorganisms is recommended to establish a positive balance of the population of useful or beneficial microbes in the intestinal flora [4].

HUMAN INTESTINAL MICROBIOTA

For years, the microbial community in our intestines has been referred to as the 'intestinal microflora', or sometimes just 'flora'. The term 'microflora' literally means 'small plants'. However, bacteria, viruses, yeasts and protozoa are taxonomically markedly different from plants, and consequently, the use of the alternative term 'microbiota' ('small life') has been recommended [5].

Moreover, the human intestinal microbiota is frequently discussed as if it were a defined entity. Accumulating scientific data indicate, however, that this population comprises a dynamic mixture of microbes, the composition of which differs both along the gastrointestinal tract and from lumen to mucosa. The microbiota develops over time, determined by an interplay between genetic factors, contact with the initial surrounding environment, diet and disease. As a result, every individual has a unique characteristic microbiota; even homozygotic twins differ in the composition of their microbiota [6].

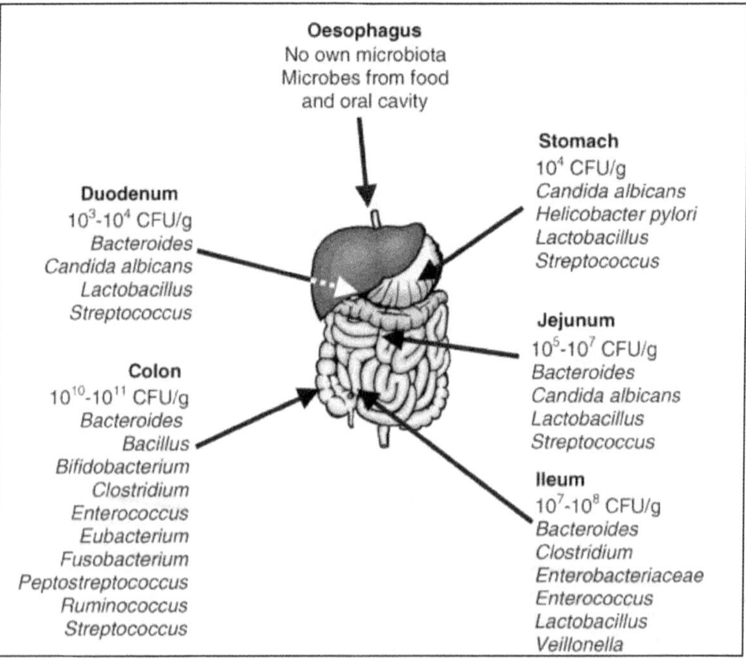

Figure 1: The numerically dominant microbial genera in the adult human gastrointestinal tract [7]

The initial compositional development of the gut microbiota

Before birth, the fetus, including its intestine, is sterile. Birth causes an abrupt end to this sterility: microbial colonization commences immediately after birth. 'Natural' delivery will expose the child to the maternal vaginal and intestinal microbiota, comprising mainly Lactobacillus, Bacteroides, Peptostreptococcus and Peptococcus, which constitute the initial source of bacteria colonizing the intestine of the newborn. Subsequently, the child will be exposed to microbes from the environment [8].

The first microbes to colonize appear to be facultative anaerobes, although strict anaerobes can also be detected from the first day of life. In any case, after 2 or 3 days anaerobes become the main microbes found in the faeces of infants. The explanation here appears to be that facultative anaerobes reduce the redox potential in the gut and render the environment suitable for obligate anaerobes [9].

Upon Caesarean section delivery, the first exposure to microbes comes directly from the environment. This altered initial exposure cannot but affect the intestinal microbiota and its development. Thus the establishment of the gut microbiota is considered a step-wise process with facultative anaerobes such as the enterobacteria, coliforms and lactobacilli first colonizing the intestine, rapidly succeeded by bifidobacteria and lactic acid bacteria . The failure of a controlled succession may culminate in the risk of developing infectious, inflammatory and allergic diseases later in life [10].

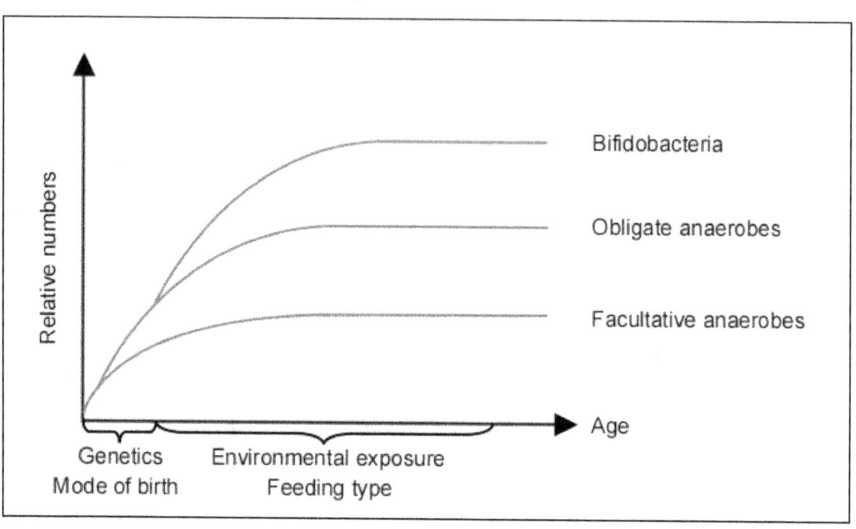

Figure 2: The establishment of the gut microbiota—a step-wise process [7]

Factors influencing the composition of the gut microbiota

The diet may exert a major effect on the composition and activity of the gut microbiota. As long as infants are breast-fed and/or formula-fed, the faecal microbiota will be dominated by bifidobacteria. Breast-feeding tends to contribute to higher levels of bifidobacteria, although with modern infant formulas the differences are now less pronounced than in the past [11]. Nevertheless, new molecular methods indicate that lactic acid-producing bacteria account for less than 1% of the total microbiota in infants, while bifidobacteria can range from 60 up to 90% of the total faecal microbiota in breast-fed infants [12,13]. The new techniques thus indicate that the greatest difference in the microbiota of breast-fed and formula-fed infant lies in the bifidobacterial composition of the intestinal microbiota, while the lactic acid bacteria composition appears to be fairly similar. With the introduction of solid foods, the microbiota undergoes a more dramatic change and becomes diverse. This diversity results in an adult-like microbiota approximately by the age of 2 [12].

Because the environment changes along the gastrointestinal tract, different microbes are found at different sites . The high flow of the contents in the upper part of the gastrointestinal tract does not allow for the accumulation of a large microbiota, and secretions from the stomach, liver and pancreas further contribute to this end. In the lower part of the gastrointestinal tract, the flow of the digesta becomes slower and its composition is less antimicrobial, supporting the establishment of a larger microbiota. Because of the anaerobicity of the lower gastrointestinal tract, anaerobic microbes start to outnumber the aerobic [14].

During adult life, the intestinal microbiota is relatively stable [15]. In old age, however, changes again take place. Levels of Bifidobacterium tend to decrease and the diversity of the Bifidobacterium microbiota tends to wane [16,17]. Despite the differences in composition, however, no significant differences in metabolic activity of the faecal microbiota between children, adults and the elderly have been observed [18].

Functions Of Intestinal Microbiota

The activity of the intestinal microbiota is comparable to that of the liver, our metabolically most active organ. The metabolic activity of the intestinal microbiota is involved in the fermentation of exogenous and endogenous carbon and energy sources. Fermentation of different types of oligosaccharide is beneficial to the host as it provides additional energy in the form of short-chain fatty acids. Of these, butyric acid, as a main energy source for the intestinal epithelium, is important in maintaining mucosal health in the colon [19]. Furthermore, several members of the intestinal microbiota produce vitamins. However, the intestinal microbiota can also utilize other substrates such as proteins and amino acids. Fermentation of these may lead to the production of a variety of toxic substances such as tumour inducers and promoter [20].

Another important function of the intestinal microbiota is to provide protection against incoming microbes. Studies have demonstrated that animals bred in a germ-free environment are highly susceptible to infections; thus, the intestinal microbiota is considered an important constituent in the mucosal defence barrier. The phenomenon in question is termed colonization resistance: bacteria in the gut mucosa compete for the same attachment sites as pathogenic bacteria, they use the same nutrients as these bacteria, and bacteria present in

the gut produce several compounds inhibiting the growth of pathogens and other transient incoming bacteria
which are not members of the residing intestinal microbiota [21].

Finally, the intestinal microbiota provides an important stimulus for the maturation of the immune system.
At birth, the immune system is immature and develops upon exposure to microbes; the number of Peyer's
patches and immunoglobulin (Ig) A producing cells increases in their presence, thereby promoting the
immunological barrier of the gut mucosa [22].

POSTBIOTICS, PREBIOTICS AND SYNBIOTICS

POSTBIOTICS

Postbiotics and can be defined as non-viable bacterial products or metabolic byproducts from probiotic microorganisms that have biologic activity in the host [19]. General, postbiotics include bacterial metabolic byproducts, such as bacteriocins, organic acids, ethanol, diacetyl, acetaldehydes and hydrogen peroxide, but it is also found that certain heat-killed probiotics can also retain important bacterial structures that may exert biological activity in the host [20].

Research shows that these metabolic products have a broad inhibitory property toward pathogenic microbes and, therefore, can be used as an alternative to antibiotics [21]. Postbiotics are non-toxic, non-pathogenic and resistance to hydrolysis by mammalian enzymes, as these are non-viable bacterial products or metabolic byproducts from probiotics.

In some instances, postbiotics can also enhance barrier function against species like Saccharomyces boulardii, and improve angiogenesis in vitro and in vivo in epithelial cells by activation of a2b1 integrin collagen receptors [22]. Similar properties have also been identified in several other probiotic species of Bifidobacterium breve, Bifidobacterium lactis, Bifidobacterium infantis, Bacteroides fragilis, Lactobacillus, Escherichia coli and Faecalibacterium prausnitzii [23].

PREBIOTICS

The term prebiotics was introduced by Gibson and Roberfroid in 1995 to describe food supplements that are non-digestible by the host but are able to exert beneficial effects by selective stimulation of growth or activity of microorganisms that are present in the intestine [23].FAO/WHO defines prebiotics as a non-viable food component that confer health benefit(s) on the host associated with modulation of the microbiota [24].

Prebiotics are a collection of nutritionally enriched compounds grouped together with the efficiency to enhance and support the growth and sustenance of specific beneficial gut microflora [25]. In general, it can be said that prebiotics is those compounds that are non-digestible and able to specifically modulate the sustenance of health-promoting gut bacteria.

They are certain nutrients that modify the gut microbial flora and have a selective role in stimulation of growth or activity of beneficial bacterial species in the gut [26,27]. Some of the common known prebiotics includes bifidogenic properties of insulin,oligofructose, and fructo-oligosaccharides (FOS) synthetically produced from sucrose, as well as galactose containing and xylose-containing oligosaccharides [28,29]. The fermentation of carbohydrates represents a major source of energy for epithelial cells in the colon and prebiotics can readily fulfill these requirements as a result of their fermentation by gut microbiota, such as bifidobacteria.

Prebiotics can be obtained naturally from sources like vegetables, fruits, and grains consumed in our daily life. They not only serve as an energy source but also have several health benefits such as reducing the prevalence and duration of diarrhea, providing relief from inflammation and other symptoms associated with intestinal bowel disorders, and exerting protective effects to prevent colon cancer [30]. They are also implicated in enhancing the bioavailability and uptake of minerals, lowering of some risk factors for cardiovascular disease, and promoting satiety and weight loss [24]. Despite their vast nutritional and medicinal benefits, research regarding screening new versatile prebiotics is scarce.

Desirable attributes	Properties of oligosaccharides
Active at low dosage	Selectively and efficiently metabolized by Bifidobacterium and / or Lactobacillus species.
Lack of side effects	Selectively and efficiently metabolized by beneficial bacteria without producing gas.
Persistence through the colon	Preferably high molecular weight
Varying viscosity	Available in different molecular weights and linkages
Acceptable storage and processing stability	Possess 1–6 linkages and pyranosyl sugar rings
Ability to control microflora modulation	Selectively metabolized by restricted microbial species.
Varying sweetness	Varying monosaccharide composition

Table 1: Properties of an ideal prebiotic [31]

Recent advancements and utility prebiotics:

Like probiotics, prebiotics is also being widely explored for their utility in the various field of applied science, more specifically as nutrients and supplements. The food industries of the present decade require simple, sustainable, cost-effective and high efficient methods for large-scale production and application. Naturally, prebiotic oligosaccharides could be obtained from food; otherwise, theses could also be synthesized chemically or enzymatically from disaccharides or other substrates as well as by hydrolysis of polysaccharides. Most of the prebiotics of natural origin have already been evaluated for their beneficiary role; therefore the current search is for other novel prebiotic oligosaccharides by various enzyme-based technologies. Enzymes (b galactosidase, fructosyltransferase etc.) from various sources such as microbes and plants are being utilized for their synthesis [32,33]. Due to the tangible association of prebiotics oligosaccharides with the gut microbiome as well as maintenance and restoration of microbial homeostasis which is again keenly associated with positive health outcome of the host, researches regarding prebiotics are given much emphasis in the current era.

Prebiotic compounds are food-grade substances from which beneficial short-chain fatty acid could be produced as a result of degradation by microbes such as bifidobacteria and lactobacilli within the host further appeal for their utilization as nutrient supplements [34]. Their biomedical benefaction not only covers gastrointestinal system but also systems located away. Recent studies several rat models have demonstrated calcium absorption, retention bone density and strength is enhanced due to the intake of galactooligosaccharides (GOS) specifically [35].It has also been found that prebiotics such as oligofructose, b-fructan, oligofructose/inulin mix have immunomodulatory benefits in the case of pathogenic attack, atopic dermatitis, allergic prevention, chronic inflammation and up-regulated responses against vaccinations [35,36].

	Bioactive compounds	Natural sources
Postbiotics		
	Bacteriocins	Lactobacillus plantarum I-UL4
	Heat-killed LGG	Lactobacillus rhamnosus
	Soluble mediator	Lactobacillus paracasei
	Butyrate	Faecalibacterium prausnitzii
	Polyphosphate	Lactobacillus brevis
	Exopolysaccharides	Lactobacillus pentosus
	Short-chain fatty acids	Lactobacillus gasser
Prebiotics		

	Fructo-oligosaccharides	Onion, Leek, Asparagus, Chicory, Jerusalem artichoke, Garlic, Wheat, Oat
	Inulin	Agave, Banana/Plantain, Burdock Camas, Chicory, Coneflower, Costus, Dandelion, Elecampane, Garlic, Globe artichoke, Jerusalem artichoke, Jicama, Leopard's bane, Mugwort root, Onion, Wild yam, Yacon
	Isomalto-oligosaccharides	Miso, Soy, Sauce, Sake, Honey
	Lactulose	Skim milk
	Lactosucrose	Milk sugar
	Galacto-oligosaccharides	Lentil, Human milk, Chickpea/hummus, Green pea, Lima bean, Kidney bean
	Soybean oligosaccharides	Soybean
	Xylo-oligosaccharides	Bamboo shoot, Fruits, Vegetables, Milk, Honey
	Fructo-oligosaccharides	Onion, Chicory, Garlic, Asparagus, Banana, Artichoke
	Arabinoxylan	Bran of grasses
	Arabinoxylan oligosaccharides	Cereals
	Resistant starch-1,2,3,4	Beans/legumes, Starchy fruits and vegetables (e.g. bananas), Whole grains

Table 2: Postbiotics, Prebiotics And Their Natural Sources [37]

SYNBIOTICS

When Gibson introduced the concept of prebiotics he speculated as to the additional benefits if prebiotics were combined with probiotics to form what he termed as Synbiotics [38].

Synbiotics is a fusion of probiotics and prebiotics products and helps in enhancing the survival and the implantation of live microbial dietary supplements in the gut [39]. The synergistic benefits are more efficiently promoted when both the probiotic and prebiotic work together in the living system. There is mounting scientific evidence that the symbiotic relationship between prebiotics and probiotics contributes significantly to health.

Synbiotics were developed to overcome possible survival difficulties for probiotics. It appears that the rationale to use synbiotics, is based on observations showing the improvement of survival of the probiotic bacteria during the passage through the upper intestinal tract. A more efficient implantation in the colon as well as a stimulating effect of the growth of probiotics and ubiquitous bacteria contribute to maintain the intestinal homeostasis and a healthy body[30]. Several factors like pH, H2O2, organic acids, oxygen, moisture stress etc. have been claimed to affect the viability of probiotics especially in dairy products like yogurts [40].

The health benefits claimed by synbiotics consumption by humans include:

1) Increased levels of lactobacilli and bifidobacteria and balanced gut microbiota,

2) Improvement of liver function in cirrhotic patients,

3) Improvement of immunomodulating ability,

4) Prevention of bacterial translocation and reduced incidences of nosocomial infections in surgical patients, etc. [41].

Prebiotics	Probiotics
Fructo-oligosaccharides	Bifidobacteria, Bacteroides fragilis, Peptostreptococcaceae, Klebsiellae
Inulin	Bifidobacterium animalis, Lactobacillus acidophilus, Lactobacillus paracasei
Isomalto-oligosaccharides	Bifidobacteria, Bacteroides fragilis group
Lactulose	Bifidobacteria lactis, Lactobacillus bulgaricus, L. acidophilus, L. rhamnosus
Lactosucrose	Zymomonas mobilis

Xylo-oligosaccharides	Bifidobacterium adolescentis, L. plantarum
Galacto-oligosaccharides	Bifidobacterium longum, B. catenulatum
Fructo-oligosaccharides	Bifidobacterium bififidum, B. lactis
Arabinoxylan and Arabinoxylan oligosaccharides	Bifidobacterium sp.
Resistant starch-1,2,3,4	Bacteroides, Eubacterium rectal

Table 3: Common Synbiotics And Their Microbial Sources [37]

DEFINITION OF PROBIOTICS

Fuller [42]: "Probiotics are live microbial feed supplements which beneficially affect the host animal by improving microbial balance".

Lilly and Stillwell [43] in 1965: Substances secreted by one microorganism that stimulate the growth of another'.

Parker in 1974 [44]: 'Organisms and substances which contribute to intestinal microbial balance'.

Salminen et al. [45]: 'Food which contains live bacteria beneficial to health'.

Marteau et al in 2002 [46]: 'microbial cell preparations or components of microbial cells that have a beneficial effect on the health and well-being'.

Charteris et al. [47]: 'microorganisms which, when ingested, may have a positive effect in the prevention and treatment of a specific pathologic condition'.

Food and Agriculture Organization of the United Nations World Health Organization: "live microorganisms which when administered in adequate amounts confer a health benefit on the host." In relation to food the definition can be adjusted by emphasizing that the beneficial effect is exerted by the microorganisms "when consumed in adequate amounts as part of food" [48].

HISTORY OF PROBIOTICS

The origin of cultured dairy products dates back to the dawn of civilization; they are mentioned in the Bible and the sacred books of Hinduism. Climatic conditions for sure favoured the development of many of the traditional soured milk or cultured dairy products such as kefir, koumiss, leben and dahi [49]. These products, many of which are still widely consumed, had often been used therapeutically before the existence of bacteria was recognized [50].

Ilya Ilyich Metchnikoff, the Nobel prize winner in Medicine in 1908, at the Pasteur Institute linked the health and longevity to ingestion of bacteria present in yoghurt [51,52]. He believed that the constitution of the human body presented several disharmonies inherited from primitive mammals, such as body hair, wisdom teeth, stomach, vermiform appendix, caecum, and large intestine. In 1907, he postulated that the bacteria involved in yoghurt fermentation, Lactobacillus bulgaricus and Streptococcus thermophilus, suppress the putrefactive-type fermentations of the intestinal flora and that consumption of these yoghurts played a role in maintaining health. Indeed, he attributed the long life of Bulgarian peasants to their intake of yoghurt containing Lactobacillus species [52]. In particular, he reported that the large intestine, useful to mammals in managing rough food composed of bulky vegetables, is useless in humans. Moreover, it is the site of dangerous intestinal putrefaction processes which can be opposed by introducing lactobacilli into the body, displacing toxin-producing bacteria, promoting health and prolonging life [53].

However, the breakthrough was achieved more than a century ago when Henry Tissier observed that gut microbiota from healthy breast fed infants were dominated by rods with a bifid shape (bifidobacteria) which were absent from formula fed infants suffering from diarrhoea, establishing the concept that they played a role in maintaining health. His suggestions for oral administration of live organisms (bifidobacteria) to patients with diarrhea (infantile diarrhea) and help restore a healthy gut flora was a first of it kind.

At that time, many others were sceptical about the concept of bacterial therapy and questioned in particular whether the yoghurt bacteria (L. bulgaricus) were able to survive intestinal transit, colonize and convey benefits [54].

In the early 1920s, L. acidophilus milk was documented to have therapeutic effects, in particular, a settling effect on digestion [55]. It was believed that colonization and growth of these microorganisms in the gut were essential for their efficacy, and therefore, the use of intestinal isolates was advocated.

In Japan in the early 1930s, Shirota focused his research on selecting the strains of intestinal bacteria that could survive passage through the gut and on the use of such strains to develop fermented milk for distribution in his clinic. His first product containing L. acidophilus Shirota (subsequently named L.casei Shirota) was the basis for the establishment of the Yakult Honsha company [56].

The modern definition of probiotic was put forward by Havenaar and Huisint Veld [57] as a viable mono or mixed culture of bacteria which, when applied to animal or man, affects the host beneficially by improving the properties of the indigenous flora.

CHARACTERISTICS OF IDEAL PROBIOTICS[59]

Fuller[3] in 1989 It s listed the following as features of a good probiotic.

1) It should be a strain, which is capable of exerting a beneficial effect on the host animal, e.g. increased growth or resistance to disease.

2) It should be non pathogenic and non-toxic.

3) It should be present as viable cells, preferably in large numbers.

4) It should be capable of surviving and metabolizing in the gut environment e.g. resistance to low pH, organic acids acid and bile.

5) It should be stable under storage and field conditions.

It is generally accepted that probiotic products should have a minimum concentration of 10^6 CFU/mL or gram and that a total of some 10^8 to 10^9 probiotic microorganisms should be consumed daily for the probiotic effect to be transferred to the consumer. Furthermore, the strains must be able to grow under manufacture and commercial conditions and should retain viability under normal storage conditions [60].

MECHANISMS OF PROBIOTIC ACTIVITY

Probiotics have various mechanisms of action although the exact manner in which they exert their effects is still not fully elucidated. These range from:

(i) bacteriocin and short chain fatty acid production,

(ii) lowering of gut pH,

(iii) nutrient competition to stimulation of mucosal barrier function and Immunomodulation

(iv) inducing phagocytosis and IgA secretion,

(v) modifying T-cell responses,

(vi) enhancing Th1 responses, and attenuating Th2 responses [60].

Mechanisms of interaction between probiotics and intestinal epithelial cells [67]:

(i) **Induction of the synthesis of cytoprotective heat shock proteins** : Intestinal epithelial cells (IEC), when in contact with heat, osmotic, oxidative, or other stresses, activate a system of "stress tolerance" based on the induction of heat shock proteins (hsp). Heat shock proteins in the gut include hsp25 (that stabilizes actin) and hsp72 (that prevents cell denaturation). These mechanisms help maintaining efficient tight junctions between IEC, thus promoting the function of the mucosal barrier. Probiotics in the gut induce the production of cytoprotective heat shock proteins.

(ii) **Modulation of inflammatory signaling systems in IEC** : IEC are equipped with signaling systems to activate the immune response and face a variety of stimuli. NF_kB represents the main system, which is present in the cytoplasm in its inactive form, bound to inhibitory molecules of the I_kB family. In the presence of pro-inflammatory stimuli, I_kB phosphorylates, detaches from NF_kB and, thus, allows NF_kB itself to migrate from the cytoplasm to the nucleus, activating the transcription of specific genes. Some probiotics modulate the degradation of I_kB whereas others stimulate NF_kB to increase the secretion of specific cytokines. Lactobacillus plantarum inhibits the activity of NF_kB and the degradation of I_kB in vitro. Another molecular target modulated by probiotics is PPAR , a nuclear receptor that can regulate the level of intestinal inflammation and, in particular, may play a role in alleviating some intestinal inflammatory diseases by inhibiting the activity of NF_kB (PPAR is, indeed, present in small amounts in the IEC of patients with inflammatory bowel disease, or IBD). Treatment with specific strains of probiotics can increase the expression of PPAR and, thereby, improve inflammation in patients with IBD.

(iii) **Regulation of apoptosis**: Some probiotics may regulate apoptosis of IEC. Lactobacillus rhamnosus GG ATCC 53103 can activate a protein with anti-apoptotic action and inhibit a protein with pro-apoptotic action in IEC stimulated with various cytokines (TNF- , IL- 1 or IFN). Some experiments show that LGG activates the production of two proteins, p75 and p40, which promote cell proliferation and activate Akt anti-apoptotic protein. The ability of probiotics to regulate apoptosis may also represent a useful strategy for the control of intestinal infections.

(iv) **Modulation of the signaling systems of macrophages** : At the gut level, probiotics modulate different signaling systems of macrophages, with effects on mucosal immunity.

Oelschlaeger reported that the effects of probiotics may be classified in three modes of action:
(i) Probiotics might be able to modulate the host's defences including the innate as well as the acquired immune system. This mode of action is most likely important for the prevention and therapy of infectious diseases but also for the treatment of (chronic) inflammation of the digestive tract or parts thereof. In addition, this probiotic action could be important for the eradication of neoplastic host cells;

(ii) Probiotics can also have a direct effect on other microorganisms, commensal and/or pathogenic ones. This principle is in many cases of importance for the prevention and therapy of infections and restoration of the microbial equilibrium in the gut;

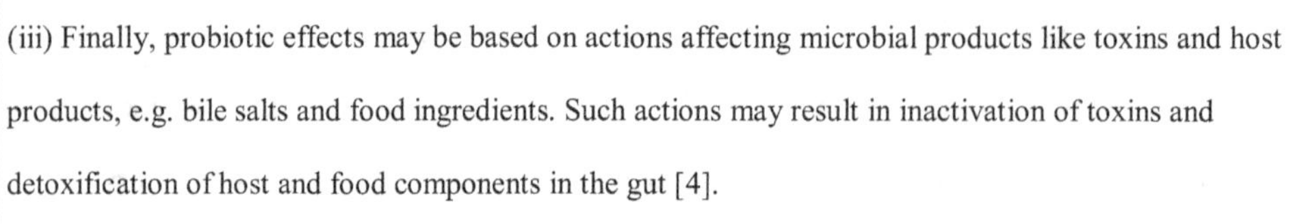

(iii) Finally, probiotic effects may be based on actions affecting microbial products like toxins and host products, e.g. bile salts and food ingredients. Such actions may result in inactivation of toxins and detoxification of host and food components in the gut [4].

The kind of effect(s) a certain probiotic executes depends on its metabolic properties, the molecules presented at its surface or on the components secreted. Even integral parts of the bacterial cell such as DNA or peptidoglycan might be of importance for its probiotic effectiveness. The individual combination of such properties in a certain probiotic strain determines a specific probiotic action and as a consequence its effective application for the prevention and/or treatment of a certain disease [4].

DRUG INTERACTIONS

Since probiotics contain live microorganisms, concurrent administration of antibiotics could kill a large number of the organisms, reducing the efficacy of the Lactobacillus and Bifidobacterium species. Patients should be instructed to separate administration of antibiotics from these bacteria-derived probiotics by at least two hours [62,63]. Similarly, S. boulardii might interact with antifungals, reducing the efficacy of this probiotic [64].

Probiotics should also be used cautiously in patients taking immunosuppressants, such as cyclosporine, tacrolimus, azathioprine, and chemotherapeutic agents, since probiotics could cause an infection or pathogenic colonization in immunocompromised patients [62,63,64].

BENEFITS OF PROBIOTIC INTERVENTION

Correction of the properties of an unbalanced indigenous microbiota forms the rationale of probiotic therapy. The benefit of manipulation of the gut microbiota here lies in cessation of the vicious circle in inflammation, clinically manifested as control of disease activity and a shortening of the duration of symptoms. Transient colonization may be important and sufficient, as unbalanced intestinal microbiota in such conditions can be corrected by brief probiotic intervention [7]

One plausible hypothesis is that the normal microbiota acquired during and immediately after delivery is needed for the development of the systemic and mucosal immunity of the newborn. An increasing number of clinical and experimental studies demonstrate that constituents within the intestinal lumen, in particular the resident microbiota, may steer the inflammatory responses in allergic and inflammatory bowel diseases. If this conception proves correct, probiotic bacteria may counteract such inflammatory process by stabilizing the gut microbial environment and the intestine's permeability barrier, and by enhancing the degradation of enteral antigens and altering their immunogenicity [7]

The window of opportunity lies in early infancy, as the first expression of the allergic disease type frequently occurs within the first months of life. The same would appear to hold true for the maturation of the gut immune defence mechanisms. Vaginally born infants and infants born by caesarean section show major differences in culturable microbiota, still to be observed at 6 months of age 5, when a substantial proportion of children born by caesarean section were not colonized with Bacteroides fragilis. Colonization appeared to be associated with the maturation of humoral immune mechanisms. Interestingly, Bacteroides fragilis and, to a lesser extent, Bifidobacterium species were important in this respect, as infants harbouring these organisms had more circulating IgA and IgM-secreting cells. These results suggest that the intestinal microbiota is important in immune regulation in human individuals, and that qualitative differences in the composition of the gut microbiota might affect the immunologic homeostasis [7].

THE RISKS OF PROBIOTIC INTERVENTION

The probiotics currently used have been assessed safe in fermented foods, but generally the safety evaluation of microbial food supplements remains to be developed. Recent species and strain assessment has focused on probiotic bacteria used in food fermentation. The ability of specific probiotic strains to survive gastric conditions and to adhere strongly to the intestinal mucosa following oral administration may entail a risk of bacterial translocation, bacteraemia and sepsis. For current probiotic foods such risks have been reported rarely, but some cases of bacteraemia in subjects especially with serious underlying diseases are known. A study from Finland summarizes a decade of rapidly increasing probiotic consumption without increases in cases of bacteraemia associated with lactic acid bacteria. It is also of importance to assess the long-term effects of probiotics administered at birth and during breast-feeding, as their oral administration may influence the development of the intestinal microbiota in newborns and the long-term effects of this are not known [7].

Effect	Potential mechanism	Potential risks
Nutritional management of acute diarrhoea	Reduction in the duration of rotavirus shedding, normalization of gut permeability and microbiota	Risk related to host and strain characteristics
Nutritional management of allergic disease Inflammatory bowel disease	Degradation/structural modification of enteral antigens, normalization of the properties of aberrant indigenous microbiota and of gut barrier functions, local and systemic inflammatory response, increase in the expression mucins	Strains with pro-inflammatory effects/adverse effects on innate immunity Translocation/infection
Reducing the risk of infectious disease	Increase in IgA-secreting cells against rotavirus, the expression of mucins	Risk related to host and strain characteristics
Reducing the risk of allergic/inflammatory disease	Promotion of gut barrier functions, anti-inflammatory potential, regulation of the secretion of inflammatory mediators, and promotion of development of the immune system	Directing the microbiota towards other adverse outcomes/directing the immune responder type to other adverse outcomes

Table 4: Potential risks of probiotic intervention

SAFETY OF PROBIOTICS

Probiotics are live micro-organisms and hence, it is possible that they may result in infection in the host. Different strains of probiotics have different safety profiles. Although probiotic therapy is generally considered safe, the concept of willingly ingesting live bacteria remains somewhat counter intuitive[65].

In theory, probiotics may be responsible for four types of side effects in susceptible individuals: systemic infections, deleterious metabolic activities, excessive immune stimulation, and gene transfer. In practice, however, lactobacilli and bifidobacteria (and probiotics based on these organisms) are extremely rare causes of infections in humans. This lack of pathogenicity extends across all age groups and also to immuno-compromised individuals [4].

Traditional dairy strains of lactic acid bacteria (LAB) have a long history of safe use. LAB, including different species of Lactobacillus and Enterococcus, have been consumed daily since humans started to use fermented milk as food. Probiotic species such as Lactobacillus acidophilus have been safely used for more than 70 years.Members of the genera Lactococcus and Lactobacillus are most commonly given the GRAS status, whilst members of the genera Streptococcus, Enterococcus and some other genera of LAB are considered opportunistic pathogens [4].

Although no serious adverse events have been described in clinical trials, systemic infections associated with specific probiotics have been noted in isolated reports. These include sepsis or endocarditis with lactobacilli, fungemia with S. boulardii, and liver abscess with LGG. Bacteremia due to lactobacilli rarely occurs, but predisposing factors include immunosuppression, prior hospitalization, severe underlying co-morbidities, previous antibiotic therapy, and prior surgical interventions. There have been several documented cases of fungemia associated with use of S. boulardii. Those at greatest risk include critically ill or highly immunocompromised patients or those with central venous catheters in place. When S. boulardii capsules are opened at the bedside for administration through the nasogastric tube, central venous catheters may become contaminated and serve as the source of entry for the organism [66].

In a review of the literature, Boyle et al. identified major and minor risk factors for probiotic-associated sepsis. Major risk factors included immunosuppression (including a debilitated state or malignancy) and prematurity in infants. Minor risk factors were the presence of a central venous catheter, impairment of the intestinal epithelial barrier (such as with diarrheal illness), cardiac valvular disease (Lactobacillus probiotics only), concurrent administration with broad-spectrum antibiotics to which the probiotic is resistant, and administration of probiotics via a jejunostomy tube (this method of delivery could increase the number of viable probiotic organisms reaching the intestine by bypassing the acidic contents of the stomach). The authors recommended that probiotics be used cautiously in patients with one major risk factor or more than one minor risk factor [66].

Three approaches can be used to assess the safety of a probiotic strain:
(i) studies on the intrinsic properties of the strain,
(ii) studies on the pharmacokinetics of the strain (survival, activity in the intestine, dose–response relation ships, faecal and mucosal recovery) and
(iii) studies searching for interactions between the strain and the host [4].

In the food sector, the introduction of new rules has also led to the adoption of new instruments for the evaluation of probiotics, based on the so-called "Qualified Presumption of Safety (QPS)" [54]. Consequently, every microbial strain for which an identity has been unequivocally established and classified in a QPS group, i.e. a group that does not raise concern from the point of view of safety, is only subjected to the verification of the absence of specific "qualifications" that may cause concern for public health before the final approval of its safety standards of use [67].

The Scientific Committee on Animal Nutrition of the EU (SCAN) and the EFSA Panel on additives, products and substances used in animal feed (FEEDAP) require the absence of transferable antibiotic resistant genes as a prerequisite for approval of a microorganism. Although there are no legally mandatory criteria for probiotics in food supplements for humans, the verification of the absence of transferable resistance is recommended for safety assessment at EU level [67].

A Working Group was convened by FAO/WHO to generate guidelines and recommend criteria and methodology for the evaluation of probiotics, and to identify and define what data need to be available to accurately substantiate health claims. The aims of the Working Group were to identify and outline the minimum requirements needed for probiotic status [50].

FAO/WHO developed Operating Standards in 2002, which gave guidelines for all companies producing probiotic products [68].

These guidelines include:

1) Implementation of guidelines for use of probiotics;

2) Phase I, II and III clinical trials to prove health benefits that are as good as or better than standard prevention or treatments for a particular condition or disease;

3) Good manufacturing practice and production of high quality products;

4) Studies to identify mechanism of action in-vivo;

5) Informative/precise labeling;

6) Development of probiotic organism that can carry vaccines to hosts and /or antiviral probiotics;

7) Expansion of proven strains to benefit the oral cavity, nasopharynx, respiratory tract, stomach, vagina, bladder and skin as well as for cancer, allergies and recovery from surgery/injury.[68]

PRECAUTION AND CONTRAINDICATIONS OF PROBIOTICS

Since probiotics contain live microorganisms, there is a slight chance that these preparations might cause pathological infection, particularly in critically ill or severely immuno-compromised patients. Probiotic strains of Lactobacillus have also been reported to cause bacteremia in patients with short-bowel syndrome, possibly due to altered gut integrity. Caution is also warranted in patients with central venous catheters, since contamination leading to fungemia has been reported when Saccharomyces capsules were opened and administered at the bedside.Lactobacillus preparations are contraindicated in persons with a hypersensitivity to lactose or milk. S. boulardii is contraindicated in patients with a yeast allergy. No contraindications are listed for bifidobacteria, since most species are considered non-pathogenic and non-toxigenic [66].

PROBIOTIC MICROORGANISMS

The probiotic potential of different bacterial strains, even within the same species, differs. Different strains of the same species are always unique, and may have differing areas of adherence (site-specific), specific immunological effects, and actions on a healthy vs. an inflamed mucosal milieu may be distinct from each other. According to Shah [69] and Chow [70] the most popular strains are represented by the following genera: Lactobacillus, Streptococcus, and Bifidobacterium, but other organisms including enterococci and yeasts have also been used as probiotics.

S.No	Probiotic bacterial genera	Species involved
1	Lactobacillus	L. plantarum, L. paracasei, L. acidophilus, L. casei, L. rhamnosus, L. crispatus, L. gasseri, L. reuteri, L. bulgaricus
2	Propionibacterium	P. jensenii, P. freudenreichii
3	Peptostreptococcus	P. Productus
4	Bacillus	B. coagulans, B. subtilis, B. laterosporus
5	Lactococcus	L. lactis, L. reuteri, L. rhamnosus, L. casei, L. acidophilus, L. curvatus, L. plantarum
6	Enterococcus	E. Faecium
7	Pediococcus	P. acidilactici, P. pentosaceus
8	Streptococcus	S. sanguis, S. oralis, S. mitis, S. thermophilus, S. salivarius
9	Bifidobacterium	B. longum, B. catenulatum, B. breve, B. animalis, B. bififidum
10	Bacteroides	B. uniformis
11	Akkermansia	A. muciniphila
12	Saccharomyces	S. boulardii

Table 5: Current Microorganisms Used As Probiotics [71]

The genus Bifidobacterium:

Bifidobacteria were first isolated and described in 1899–1900 by Tissier, who described rod-shaped, non-gas-producing, anaerobic microorganisms with bifidobacterial morphology, present in the faeces of breast-fed infants, which he termed Bacillus bifidus. Bifidobacteria are generally characterized as Gram-positive, non-spore-forming, non-motile and catalase-negative anaerobes [72]. They have various shapes including short, curved rods, club-shaped rods and bifurcated Y-shaped rods. Presently, 30 species are included in the genus Bifidobacterium, 10 of which are from human sources (dental caries, faeces and vagina), 17 from animal intestinal tracts or rumen, two from wastewater and one from fermented milk [73].

Bifidobacteria are microorganisms of paramount importance in the active and complex ecosystem of the intestinal tract of humans and other warm-blooded animals, as well as of honeybees [72]. They are distributed in various ecological niches in the human gastrointestinal and genitourinary tracts, the exact ratio of which is determined mainly by the age and diet. The indigenous microflora of infants is dominated by bifidobacteria, which are established shortly after birth. Their proliferation is stimulated by the glycoprotein components of k-casein in human colostrum and, to a lesser extent, human milk. The number of bifidobacteria decreases with increasing age of an individual and eventually becomes the third most abundant genus (accounting for approx. 25 % of the total adult gut flora) after the genera Bacteroides and Eubacterium [74].

The genus Lactobacillus

In 1990, Moro was the first researcher to isolate a strain which he typified as Bacillus acidophilus, a generic name for intestinal lactobacilli. Lactobacilli are in general characterized as Gram-positive, non-spore-forming and non-flagellated rods or coccobacilli [75]. They are either aerotolerant or anaerobic and strictly fermentative. Glucose is fermented predominantly to lactic acid in the homofermentative case, or equimolar amounts of lactic acid, CO2 and ethanol (and/or acetic acid) in the heterofermentative counterpart. Gomes and Malcata [73] reported that 56 species of the genus Lactobacillus have been recognized. Lactobacilli are distributed in various ecological niches throughout the gastrointestinal and genital tracts and constitute an important part of the indigenous microflora of man and higher animals. Their distribution is affected by several environmental factors, which include pH, oxygen availability, level of specific substrates, presence of secretions and bacterial interactions. They are rarely associated with cases of gastrointestinal and extraintestinal infection, and strains employed technologically are regarded as non-pathogenic and safe microorganisms. Furthermore, they have the reputation of health promoters, especially in the human gastrointestinal and genitourinary tracts [76].

Other probiotic microorganisms

Although the term probiotic is more related to lactic acid bacteria as Lactobacillus and Bifidobacterium, it can be extended to other microorganisms which have not been explored. For example, Bacillus species have been used as probiotics for at least 50 years in an Italian product commercialized as Enterogermina® ($2 \cdot 10^9$ spores). Among this group some species that have been evaluated are Bacillus subtilis, Bacillus clausii, Bacillus cereus, Bacillus coagulans and Bacillus licheniformis [77]. Some advantages of the bacterial spores are their resistance to heat, allowing the storage at room temperature and in a dried form. Also, these bacteria are able to reach small intestine since they survive the gastric pH of the stomach [78]. The application of probiotic bacterial spores ranges from dietary supplements to growth promoters and uses in aquaculture (e.g. shrimp) [77].

Probiotic formulations involving some Bacillus species are recommended for use with antibiotics since these strains are resistant to them (e.g. B. clausii) [79]. B. coagulans has been used as adjunct therapy for relieving rheumatoid arthritis [80]. B. subtilis has been researched genetically and physiologically, and is strongly associated with a Japanese product known as natto. The consumption of this product can lead to stimulation of the immune system and reduction of blood coagulation by fybrinolysis [81,82]. The secretion of antimicrobials such as coagulin, amicoumacin and subtilisin is also verified in Bacillus.

The proposed mechanisms for probiotic effects of the Bacillus spores are based on immunomodulation, which occurs through the stimulation of the gut-associated lymphoid tissue (GALT) by production of cytokines, competitive exclusion of gastrointestinal pathogens (e.g. competition for adhesion sites) and secretion of antimicrobial substances [83].

Several studies have been performed to assure the safety of Bacillus species using animal models and in vitro tests to evaluate the toxicity or adverse effects of the strains. The use of B. subtilis is approved for use as a supplement in Italy and the UK. However, the designation 'probiotic' should only be allowed if the microorganism presents the characteristics inherent to probiotic strains. On the other hand, studies of competitive exclusion of Escherichia coli 078:K80 by Bacillus subtilis [84] and the suppression of Vibrio harveyi in shrimp by several Bacillus spore formers [85] have strongly shown the probiotic potential of these strains.

Probiotic microorganisms used in animal preparations are Enterococcus, Bacillus, Streptococcus, Lactobacillus, Aspergillus and Saccharomyces [86]. Vitacanis® is a probiotic formulation which can be used in preventing intestinal disorders in dogs and cats. Among Enterococcus species, Enterococcus faecium is the most used in commercial probiotics. The presence of Enterococcus faecium is important in preventing infection by Salmonella enterica ssp. enterica ser. Typhimurium [87]. Additionally, a probiotic product known as Causido®, which contains S. thermophilus and E. faecium, has been proposed for a short-term hypocholesterolaemic effect [88]. Interesting characteristics of the Enterococcus group are the survival on dry surfaces for prolonged periods and the resistance to antibiotics [89].

Among the probiotic yeasts, the most common genus is Saccharomyces, which has been employed in livestock feed. S. cerevisiae has shown a beneficial effect when administrated in the Nile tilapia as growth promoter [90]. The potential probiotic effect of S. cerevisiae and S. cerevisiae var. boulardii has been demonstrated since they are able to tolerate low pH and bile and protect against bacterial infections through the reduction of the intestinal pro-inflammatory response [91]. However, the adhesion properties of these yeasts should be better investigated.

QUANTIFICATION OF PROBIOTICS

Traditionally, appropriate dilutions of faecal samples have been cultured on selective media. However, the selectivity of any medium is at best relative and these methods are prone to both false-positive and false-negative results. More importantly, not all microbes can be cultured by the currently available techniques. With the advent of molecular biology, culture-independent techniques have been developed. In particular,methods using the variable and conserved regions of the 16S rRNA have proved successful in characterizing the gut microbiota. The use of 16S rRNA enables enumeration of microbes which are either unculturable by the current cultivation techniques or have died during transport and storage. Fluorescent in situ hybridization (FISH) is commonly used and employs species-, genusor domain-specific fluorescently labelled 16S rRNA probes. Enumeration of the labelled microbes can be done microscopically by visual counting, which is, however, laborious. On the other hand, although image analysis of the microscopic view makes it possible to process a relatively large number of samples, this is expensive. Alternatively, enumeration of fluorescent microbes can be done by flow cytometry, which similarly allows the analysis of large numbers of samples, but is also expensive. Techniques based on the polymerase chain reaction (PCR) are also commonly used and provide rapid quantitative and qualitative information on the composition of the intestinal microbiota [4].

TECHNOLOGY OF PROBIOTICS

Probiotics are certainly very sensitive to many environmental stresses, such as acidity, oxygen and heat. Before a probiotic can benefit human health, it must fulfill several criteria related to

Safety and Stability:

(i) activity and viability in products;

(ii) adherence;

(iii) invasive potential;

(iv) resistance to low pH,

(v) gastric juice, bile acid and pancreatic juice;

(vi) colonization/survival in vivo and

Functional and Physiological aspects:

(i) adherence to intestinal epithelium/tissue/virulence,

(ii) antagonism to pathogens,

(iii) antimicrobial activity,

(iv) stimulation/suppression of immune response,

(v) selective stimulation of beneficial bacteria and

(vi) clinical side effects in volunteers/patients

The viability of probiotics is a key parameter for developing probiotic foods. Several factors affect the viability of probiotic bacteria until they reach the target site of the host [92].

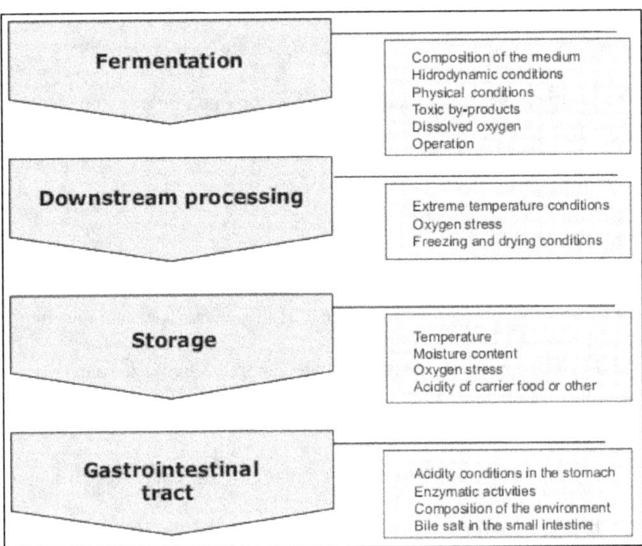

Figure 3: Factors influencing the stability of probiotics during processing steps [92]

CHALLENGE FOR PROBIOTIC FORMULATION

Inappropriate use of the term "probiotic" and failure to recognize the importance of the strain specificity and dose specificity is a concern today. Probiotics when produced as nutritional supplements, not drugs, undergo less regulatory scrutiny as it is not mandatory for the manufacturer to substantiate claims of efficacy or safety of foods and nutraceutical supplements. This is a main reason for poor to non-existent efficacy and safety information on most commercial products.

The challenge for experts working on the medical aspect of functional foods and probiotics, prebiotics, synbiotics and novel foods is to apply the new knowledge generated by basic scientists in the field of intestinal flora. Probiotic research stands today at the intersection of gastroenterology, immunology and microbiology and is highly dynamic in both the basic and the clinical field. Further understanding of the complex molecular mechanisms leading to the effectiveness of probiotics will also spur the development of more successful probiotic formulations.

The pitfalls and inherent defects of commercial probiotic products and remedial measure are delivery of inadequate quantity of probiotics to the lower gastrointestinal tract - specifically the acidic environment of the stomach. Therefore, a more specific target delivery system along with appropriate dosage needs to be evolved. Additional developments required are:

1) The probiotic formulation should have an enhanced shelf life and should deliver live active probiotic cells even after prolonged storage

2) Evaluation methods need to be established to make sure that the formulation actually contains clinically proven viable probiotics bacteria [93].

PROBIOTICS AND FOOD PRODUCTS

As it was reported by Chow , the notion that food could serve as medicine was first conceived thousands of years ago by the Greek philosopher and father of medicine, Hippocrates, who once wrote: 'Let food be thy medicine, and let medicine be thy food'. However, during recent times, the concept of food having medicinal value has been reborn as 'functional foods'. A probiotic may also be a functional food [95]. Functional foods are defined as: 'foods that contain some health-promoting component(s) beyond traditional nutrients'. Functional foods are also known as designer foods, medicinal foods, nutraceuticals, therapeutic foods, superfoods, foodiceuticals, and medifoods. In general, the term refers to a food that has been modified in some way to become 'functional'. One way in which foods can be modified to become functional is by the addition of probiotics [68].

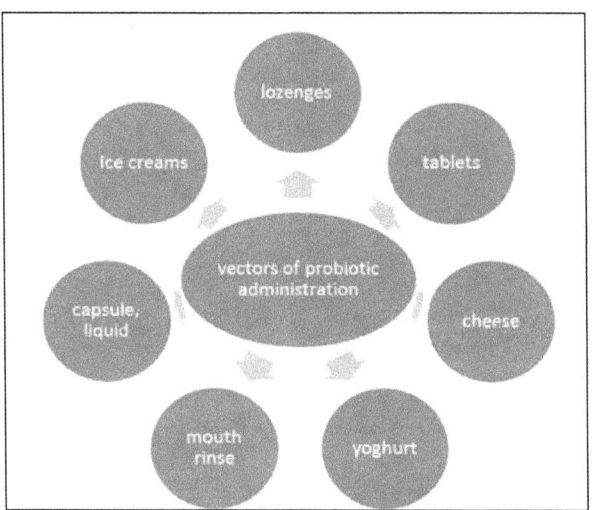

Figure 4: Probiotic Administration Methods [94]

Dairy products

The main products existing in the market are dairy-based ones including fermented milks, cheese, ice cream, buttermilk, milk powder, and yogurts, the latter accounting for the largest share of sales . Dairy products are especially considered as ideal vehicle for delivering probiotic bacteria to the human gastrointestinal tract.

The most common means to incorporate probiotics to fermented milk include:

(i) addition of probiotics together with the starter cultures (DVI culture);

(ii) the production of two batches separately, one containing the probiotic microorganism in milk to achieve a high concentration of viable cells and another with starter cultures. When the fermentation stages are completed, the batches are mixed;

(iii) the use of a probiotic microorganism as a starter culture. In this situation, the time of fermentation is generally higher than traditional processes using non-probiotic starter cultures [96].

Yoghurts with high fat content showed inhibitory effects against probiotic cultures, particularly B. bifidum BBI. The supplementation with vitamins (e.g. ascorbic acid) has been reported to improve the viability of L. acidophilus in yoghurts. The addition of substances such as whey protein may also enhance the viability of some probiotics, probably due to their buffering property[4].

The utilization of probiotics in the cheese elaboration presents some challenges:

(i) low moisture content;

(ii) presence of salt;

(iii) starter cultures competing for nutrients and developing acid and flavour during the maturation stage;

(iv) extended storage (over 3 months), which can influence biochemical activities, redox potential, and alter the cheese structure.

(v) Probiotics should survive the entire shelf life of the cheese, not produce metabolites that affect the cheese quality and the starter culture activities, and also, they should be able to grow in starter culture media (e.g. whey-based and phage inhibitory media) [4].

Other vehicles that could be used to deliver probiotics are ice cream and frozen dairy desserts. These products have the advantage to be stored at low temperatures, which makes them less exposed to abusive temperatures having higher viability at the time of consumption. Besides, they are consumed by people of all ages and are composed of milk proteins, fat and lactose as well as other compounds that are required for bacterial growth. Some prebiotics could be used to improve the characteristics of the probiotic ice creams. Inulin demonstrated to be beneficial to the firmness, melting properties and dripping time of the ice creams. Besides, the inulin level in ice cream enhanced the viability of L. acidophilus and B. lactis . The addition of oligofructose in low-fat ice cream also improved the survival of L. acidophilus La-5 and B. animalis ssp. lactis Bb-12 during storage at −18 °C for 90 days . However, to efficiently produce probiotic ice cream, it is important to select oxygen-resistant strains since the incorporation of air (overrun) in the mixture occurs in the production process, which is harmful to microaerophilic and anaerobic strains such as Lactobacillus sp. and Bifidobacterium species. This type of challenge can be resolved by the use of microencapsulation technique. As an alternative, aerated dairy dessert (e.g. chocolate mousse) has also been used as a potential agent to deliver probiotics [4].

Microencapsulation technologies:

It has been developed to protect the bacteria from damage caused by external environment. [60]. Microencapsulation is defined as a technology of packaging solids, liquids or gaseous materials in miniature, sealed capsules that can release their contents at controlled rates under the influences of specific conditions . A microcapsule consists of a semipermeable, spherical, thin, and strong membrane surrounding a solid/liquid core, with a diameter varying from a few microns to 1 mm. Encapsulation in hydrocolloid beads entraps or immobilizes the cells within the bead matrix, which in turn provides protection in such an environment . There are several techniques such as spray drying, freeze drying, fluidized bed drying for encapsulating the cultures and converting them into a concentrated powdered form. However, the bacteria encapsulated by these techniques are completely released in the product. In this case, the cultures are not protected from the product environment or during the passage through the stomach or intestinal tract[4].

Food-grade polymers such as alginate, chitosan, carboxymethyl cellulose (CMC), carrageenan, gelatin and pectin are mainly applied, using various microencapsulation technologies. The most widely used encapsulating material is alginate, a linear heteropolysaccharide of D-mannuronic and L-guluronic acids extracted from various species of algae. Alginate beads can be formed by both extrusion and emulsion methods . The use of alginate is favoured because of its low cost, simplicity, and biocompatibility. Other materials used with the emulsion technique which avoid the release of the cultures in the food product are a mixture of k-carrageenan and locust bean gum, cellulose acetate phthalate, chitosan, and gelatine [4].

Several factors, such as the capsule size, the method of microencapsulation, the coating of the capsules, the technological properties of probiotic strains with regard to processing and heat stability, the resistance of probiotic strains to the acidic conditions present in the gut, and the presumed synergistic effects of pro- and prebiotics by combining them in a single product, have been observed to strongly influence the viability of the probiotic cultures and, as a result, further research is still needed in this area [4].

Microcapsules and microspheres can be engineered to gradually release active ingredients . A microcapsule may be opened by many different means, including fracture by heat, solvation, diffusion, and pressure. A coating may also be designed to open in the specific areas of the body. A microcapsule containing acid-labile core materials that will be consumed by gastrointestinal fluids must not be fractured until after it passes through the stomach. A coating must therefore be used that is able to withstand acidic conditions in the stomach and allows active ingredients to pass through the stomach[4].

Non-dairy products

Some limitations of the use of dairy products to deliver probiotics are the presence of allergens and requirement of cold environments. This fact has led to the launch of new products based on non-dairy matrices [4].

Nondairy food applications include soy based products, nutrition bars, fruits, vegetables, legumes, cereals, and a variety of juices as appropriate means of probiotic delivery to the consumer [91]. However, the incorporation of probiotics in fruit juices requires the protection against acid conditions. This can be achieved by microencapsulation technologies, which allow the entrapment of cells into matrices with a protective coating. Gelatin and vegetable gum have been demonstrated to provide a good protection for acid-sensitive Bifidobacterium and Lactobacillus [4].

Probiotic strains usually found in vegetable materials are species belonging to Lactobacillus and Leuconostoc genera. L. plantarum, L. casei and L. delbrueckii, for example, were able to grow in cabbage juice without nutrient supplementation and reached 108 CFU/mL after 48 h of incubation at 30 oC . Inaddition, it was found that these same bacteria grew in beet juice.

In the case of cereals, the fermentation with probiotic microorganisms could be beneficial due to the decrease of nondigestible carbohydrates (poly- and oligosaccharides), the improvement of the quality and level of lysine, the availability of the vitamin B group, as well as the degradation of phytates and release of minerals (e.g. manganese, iron, zinc, and calcium). Oat-based substrates have proved promissory for the growth of L. reuteri, L. acidophilus and B. bifidum. In addition, cereals such as oats and barley contain high levels of b-glucan, which is believed to have hypocholesterolemic effect. Boza, an acid and low-alcohol beverage produced in the Balkan Peninsula, is a fermented product based on maize, wheat and other cereals. Todorov et al studied the microflora of boza and verified the presence of several lactic acid bacteria with probiotic characteristics [4].

Soybean is an important cereal because it has a high nutritive value. However, the unpleasant bean flavour and the content of oligosaccharides (e.g. stachyose and raffinose) can cause flatulence. Besides the improvement of the flavour of soybean products, fermentation can reduce flatulence, since lactic acid bacteria are able to hydrolyze a-1,6-galactosidic linkages, releasing a-D-galactose and making these products more digestible. The survival of probiotics has been assayed in soymilk and this substrate has shown to be efficient for the growth of species such as L. casei, L. acidophilus, B. infantis, and B. longum . In addition, the antioxidative activities of soymilk can be increased after fermentation by lactic acid bacteria and bifidobacteria. This has led to the designing of the probiotic soybean yoghurt [4].

Malt, wheat and barley extracts demonstrated to have a good influence in increasing bile tolerance and viability of L. acidophilus, L. reuteri and L. plantarum. Fermented foods with probiotic strains had an increment in the content of the vitamin B complex. Arora et al found an enhancement of 14 and 11 % in thiamine and niacin contents, respectively, when food mixture based on germinated barley flour with whey powder and tomato pulp were autoclaved and fermented by L. acidophilus. Also, non-germinated and germinated mixture showed an increase of 31 and 34 % in lysine content, respectively, after autoclaving and fermentation, highlighting the importance of the germination and fermentative process on the bioavailability and improvement of the nutritional quality of foods [4].

The factors that must be addressed in evaluating the effectiveness of the incorporation of the probiotic strains into such products are, besides safety, the compatibility of the product with the microorganism and the maintenance of its viability through food processing, packaging, and storage conditions. The product's pH for instance is a significant factor determining the incorporated probiotic's survival and growth, and this is one of the reasons why so cheeses seem to have a number of advantages over yoghurt as delivery systems for viable probiotics to the gastrointestinal tract [60].

DOSAGE AND PRODUCT SELECTION

Probiotics are available as supplements (i.e., tablets, capsules, or powders) and as fermented dairy products (i.e., yogurt and milk). Their efficacy relies on their ability to survive passage through the gastrointestinal tract and colonize a tissue section. For colonization to occur, probiotics must contain living, viable organisms and must be ingested on a regular basis in order to maintain effective concentrations. Unfortunately, the manufacturing process may cause living organisms to become nonviable, thus reducing probiotic effectiveness. Probiotic dosing varies depending on the product and specific indication. Products should be stored according to the manufacturer's recommendations, since some may require refrigeration. In addition, preparations may have a limited shelf life, and many preparations contain several different species, so dosing may vary depending on the product [66].

Indication and Probiotic	Recommended dosage regimen
Acute infectious diarrhea in infants and children Lactobacillus rhamnosus GG (LGG)	At least 10^{10} CFU in 250 mL of oral rehydration solution25; 10^{10}–10^{11} CFU twice daily for 2–5 days
Lactobacillus reuteri	10^{10}–10^{11} CFU daily up to 5 days
Antibiotic-associated diarrhea Saccharomyces boulardii	4×10^9 –2×10^{10} CFU daily for 1–4 wk
LGG	6×10^9 –4×10^{10} CFU daily for 1–2 wk
Lactobacillus acidophilus and Lactobacillus bulgaricus	2×10^9 CFU daily for 5–10 days
L. acidophilus and Bifidobacterium longum	5×10^9 CFU daily for 7 days
L. acidophilus and Bifidobacterium lactis	1×10^{11} CFU daily for 21 days
Clostridium difficile infection S. boulardii	2×10^{10} CFU (1 g) daily for 4 wk plus vancomycin and/or metronidazole
Travelers' diarrhea LGG	2×10^9 bacteria daily starting 2 days before departure and continued throughout trip3

S. boulardii	$5 \times 10^9 - 2 \times 10^{10}$ CFU daily starting 5 days before departure and continued throughout trip
Irritable bowel syndrome VSL#3b	9×10^{11} CFU daily for 8 wk
Bifidobacterium infantis 35624	$10^6 - 10^{10}$ CFU daily for 4 wk
LGG and other organism	$8–9 \times 10^9$ CFU daily for 6 mo
Ulcerative colitis (UC) Escherichia coli Nissle 1917	Active UC: 5×10^{10} bacteria twice daily until remission (maximum of 12 wk), followed by 5×10^{10} bacteria daily for a maximum of 12 mo39; inactive UC: 5×10^{10} bacteria daily (study duration was 12 wk
S. boulardii	Active UC: 250 mg 3 times daily for 4 wk plus mesalamine
VSL#3b	Active UC: 1.8×10^{12} bacteria (two 3-g sachets) twice daily for 6 wk plus conventional therapy
Crohn's disease S. boulardii	Maintenance therapy: 1 g daily for 6 mo plus mesalamine
Pouchitis VSL#3b	Maintenance therapy: 1.8×10^{12} bacteria daily, given as 3-g sachets twice daily (study duration was 9 mo)46; maintenance therapy: 1.8×10^{12} bacteria daily, given as two 3-g sachets once daily (study duration was 12 mo)
Atopic disease prevention LGG	10^{10} CFU daily for 2–4 wk before expected delivery in pregnant women, followed by infant administration for 6 mo
Vulvovaginal candidiasis LGG	10^9 bacteria per suppository inserted twice daily for 7 days
L. rhamnosus GR-1 and Lactobacillus fermentum RC-14	At least 10^9 bacteria suspended in skim milk given orally twice daily for 14 days
L. acidophilus	8 oz yogurt containing $\geq 10^8$ CFU/mL ingested daily for 6 mo

Table 6 : Probiotic species and dosing [66]

NEW TRENDS IN PROBIOTIC PRODUCTS AND PROCESSING

In general, consumer's understanding of the potential benefits of foods containing viable bacteria/probiotics is poor, particularly in the countries without a tradition of cultured/sour dairy products. There are many barriers to communicating messages about probiotics and the role of diet in the gut flora modulation. However, in the countries where there have been well planned educational programmes among consumers and health professionals, the degree of awareness has increased . In the future, health claims may help inform consumers of the potential benefits, but it is crucial that appropriate communication guidelines are adhered to and that all claims are scientifically substantiated [92].

Recent interest on probiotics has been stimulated by several factors:

(i) exciting scientific and clinical findings using well documented probiotic organisms;

(ii) concerns over limitations and side effects of pharmaceutical agents; and

(iii) consumer's demand for natural products.

The key to the future of probiotics will be the establishment of a consensus on product regulation, including enforcement of guidelines and standards, appropriate clinical studies that define strengths and limitations of products, and basic science studies that uncover the mechanisms of action of strains. Besides, the molecular elucidation of the probiotic actions in vivo will help to identify true probiotics and select the most suitable ones for the prevention and/or treatment of a certain illness [92].

HEALTH BENEFITS OF PROBIOTICS

There is increasing evidence in favour of the claims of beneficial effects attributed to probiotics, including improvement of intestinal health, enhancement of the immune response, reduction of serum cholesterol, and cancer prevention [60]. Among several therapeutic applications of the probiotics can be cited the prevention of urogenital diseases, alleviation of constipation, protection against traveller's diarrhoea, protection against colon and bladder cancer, prevention of osteoporosis and food allergy [97].

There is substantial evidence to support probiotic use in the treatment of acute diarrhoeal diseases, prevention of antibiotic-associated diarrhoea, and improvement of lactose metabolism, but there is insufficient evidence to recommend them for use in other clinical conditions [60].

There are several reports about the action of the probiotics against Helicobacter pylori, a Gram-negative bacterium associated with the development of chronic gastritis, peptic ulcers and gastric cancer. It was reported that L. salivarius inhibited the colonization and the release of interleukin-8 in gnotobiotic mice inoculated with H. pylori [4].

Clinical studies have suggested the efficacy of the administration of probiotics in maintaining the remission of the pouchitis, ulcerative colitis, and Crohn's disease. Patients suffering from ulcerative colitis (UC) were treated with Escherichia coli Nissle 1917 and Lactobacillus rhamnosus GG and the results were similar to that of the standard medication (5-aminosalicylic acid – Mesalazine) [4].

There is evidence that probiotic bacteria are dietary components that may play a role in decreasing cancer incidence. The exact mechanisms are under investigation, but studies have demonstrated that certain members of Lactobacillus and Bifidobacterium species decrease the levels of carcinogenetic enzymes produced by colonic flora through normalization of intestinal permeability and microflora balance as well as production of antimutagenic organic acids and enhancement of the host's immune system [60]. Roller et al correlated the inhibition of carcinogenesis in rats with changes in the immune activity, in response to probiotic consumption. Furthermore, the protective role of probiotics in rodent models of colon carcinogenesis can be found in some other studies . Studies in animal models also suggest that increasing natural killer cell activity by probiotic consumption may have potential effects on delayed tumour development [4].

Studies have also suggested that probiotics could have beneficial effects beyond some metabolic disorders such as hypertension. Primary hypertension is caused by various factors and the predominant causes include hypercholesterolemia [98]. Rising evidence has indicated that lactobacilli and bifidobacteria could cause, when ingested, a significant reduction in serum cholesterol. This is because cholesterol synthesis mainly occurs in the intestines, hence the gut microflora promote effects on lipid metabolism. Some studies demonstrated that probiotics could promote a decrease in the blood cholesterol levels and increase the resistance of low-density lipoprotein to oxidation, therefore leading to a reduced blood pressure [99].

Environment and lifestyle such as high-fat diet are some of the factors that play a key role in the development of obesity. Recent advances have identified the gut microbiota as one such environmental factor that modulates host energy and lipid metabolism [100]. Most of the data obtained have been done in experimental animal studies, but promising effects are also shown in humans, thereby supporting the interest in the nutritional modulation of the gut microbiota in the management of metabolic diseases in obese patients.[101]

Furthermore, evidence suggests that food products containing probiotic bacteria could possibly contribute to coronary heart disease prevention by reducing serum cholesterol levels as well as to blood pressure control. Probiotic strains administered in dairy products have shown to improve the therapeutic outcome in women with bacterial vaginosis, most probably by supporting the normal vaginal lactobacilli microbiota [102].

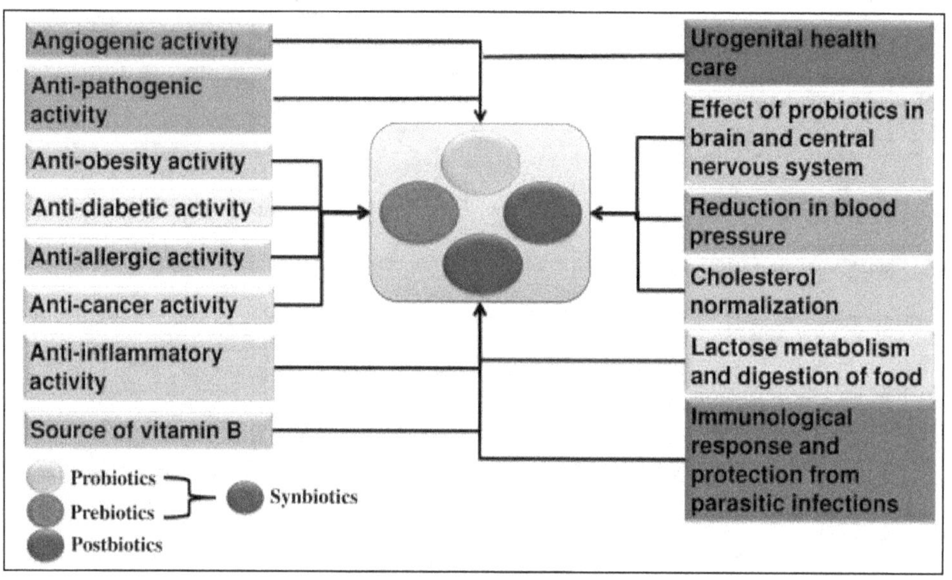

Figure 5: Application of Probiotics

1. Anti-pathogenic activity of probiotics [71]:

Anti-pathogenic activity is regarded as one of the most beneficial effects of probiotics because unlike classic antibiotics, disturbance or alteration in the composition of the complex population of the gut microbiota is inhibited.

Tejero-Sarinena et al investigated the influence of probiotics on the survival of Salmonella enterica, Serovar typhimurium and Clostridium diffificile in an in vitro model and postulated that probiotics inhibit pathogens by the production of short-chain fatty acids (SCFAs), such as acetic, propionic, butyric and lactic acids. SCFAs help to maintain an appropriate pH in the colonic lumen, which is imperative in the expression of numerous bacterial enzymes and in metabolism of foreign compounds and carcinogens in the gut.

Islam suggested that a wide variety of anti-pathogenic compounds, like bacteriocins, ethanol, organic acids, diacetyl, acetaldehydes, hydrogen peroxide (H2O2) and peptides are produced by many probiotics. Among these compounds, peptides and bacteriocins, in particular are mostly involved in increasing the membrane permeability of the target cells, which leads to the depolarization of the membrane potential and, ultimately, cell death. Similarly, the production of H_2O_2 by these bacterial groups causes the oxidation of sulfhydryl groups, resulting in the denaturation of several enzymes results in the peroxidation of membrane lipids, thus, increasing membrane permeability of the pathogenic microorganism and consequently, cell death.

Probiotics also stimulate host antipathogenic defense pathways, such as stimulating or activating the pathway involved in the production of defensins that are cationic anti-microbial peptides produced in several cell types including Paneth cells in the crypts of the small intestine and intestinal epithelial cells. Another mechanism by which probiotics exert anti-pathogenic activity is by competing for pathogen binding and receptor sites, as well as for available nutrients and growth.

2. Urogenital health care [71]:

According to the Centers for Disease Control and Prevention (CDCP), more than one billion women around the world suffer from non-sexually transmitted urogenital infections, such as bacterial vaginosis (BV), urinary tract infection (UTI) and several other yeast infections. The species typically associated with BV include Gardnerella vaginalis, Ureaplasma urealyticum, and Mycoplasma hominis. Sexually transmitted diseases (STDs) are also a significant cause of morbidity worldwide. The two most commonly documented bacterial STDs in some developed countries are gonorrhea and Chlamydia, which are caused by Neisseria gonorrhoeae and Chlamydia trachomatis, respectively.

It is well-known that there is an association between abnormal vaginal microbial flora and an increased incidence of urinary tract infection (UTI). There are about 50 different species inhabiting the vagina, like

Lactobacillus species, Lactobacillus brevis, Lactobacillus casei, Lactobacillus vaginalis, Lactobacillus delbrueckii, Lactobacillus salivarius, Lactobacillus reuteri, and Lactobacillus rhamnosus that are regarded as the main regulators of the vaginal micro-environment. Imbalance in the microbial composition greatly influences the health of the vaginal microenvironment, potentially leading to compromised state of bacterial vaginosis (BV) and UTI. These compromised states can be reassured by balancing the number of Lactobacillus sp. via the supplementation of probiotics.

3. Immune system [103]:

Evidence from in vitro systems, animal models and humans suggests that probiotics can enhance both the specific and nonspecific immune response, possibly by activating macrophages, increasing levels of cytokines, increasing natural killer cell activity, and/or increasing levels of immunoglobulins. In spite of limited testing in humans, these results may be particularly important to the elderly, who could benefit from an enhanced immune response. The immune system effects of probiotics are to enhance specific and nonspecific immune response, inhibit pathogen growth and translocation, and reduce chance of infection from common pathogens (Salmonella, Shigella).

4. Role In Prevention Of Transmission of AIDS And STDs [65]:

Lactobacilli play a critical role in the regulation of the vaginal microflora. It has been suggested that the production of H2O2 rather than a particular species of Lactobacillus, is essential in the regulation of the vaginal flora. This toxic molecule is the most potent local microbicide present in the human vagina. The findings of experiments have suggested that LB+ given at high concentrations is viricidal for HIV- 1.There is also an inverse association between vaginal Lactobacilli and HIV seroconversion. These studies suggest that LB+ may play a role in protecting women against some pathogens in the vagina.

5. Respiratory infections [67]:

Studies have shown positive effects of probiotics on the respiratory system, especially in preventing and reducing the severity of respiratory infections, due to an increase in IgA-secreting cells in the bronchial mucosa. The role of malnutrition and deficiency of some micronutrients and vitamins has also been demonstrated in the process of viral pathogens cell entry and replication. The preventive use of supplements containing substances active on the immune system plays an important role both before vaccination and as adjuvant in vaccines, to increase antibodies in the elderly and debilitated subjects.

6. Anti-hypertension [103]:

Some preliminary evidence suggests that food products derived from probiotics bacteria could possibly contribute to blood pressure control. This antihypertensive effect has been documented with studies in spontaneous hypertensive rats. Two tripeptides, valine- proline-proline and isoleucine-proline- p a milk-based medium by roline, isolated from fermentation of Saccharomyces cereviseae and Lactobacillus helveticushave been identified as the active components. These tripeptides function as angiotensin I-converting enzyme inhibitors and reduce blood pressure.

7. Children [67]:

A randomized, double-blind, placebo-controlled trial was performed to determine whether probiotics may reduce the risk of infections in infants. The children involved in the research were younger than 2 months of age and were daily provided with milk containing L. rhamnosus GG and Bifidobacterium lactis Bb-12, or placebo milk, administered until 12 months of age. The results suggest that probiotics may represent a mean to reduce the risk of early acute otitis media and the use of antibiotics for recurrent respiratory infections during the first year of life. Similar results have emerged in a study performed on a target population of 326 children aged between 3 and 5 years, showing more than 65% decrease in the incidence of antibiotic use and 25% reduction in school missed days among children treated with probiotics.

8. Adults [67]:

A randomized double-blind, placebo-controlled trial assessed whether the consumption for 3 months of Lactobacillus gasser PA 16/8, Bifidobacterium longum SP 07/3, B. bifidum MF 20/5, had impacts on symptoms severity, incidence and duration of common cold. For two winter/spring seasons, 479 adults were daily treated with vitamins and minerals enriched or not with probiotics. The results indicate a reduction in the duration of episodes of common cold of at least 2 days and a decrease in the severity of symptoms among subjects receiving probiotics if compared to the randomized placebo-control group. Similar conclusions were obtained in a study that assessed the effect of long-term intake of probiotics on the same pathology.

9. Elders [67]:

Two multicentre, randomized, controlled, double-blind studies were conducted in two successive vaccine seasons (pilot study and control). 86 and 222 elderly volunteers consumed, respectively, a fermented milk drink containing L. casei DN-114 001, a fermented yogurt or a control unfermented dairy product, twice a day for a period of 7 or 13 weeks. Vaccination took place after 4 weeks. The study showed that probiotics improve antibody responses to influenza vaccination in individuals over 70 years. L. casei DN-114001 was also evaluated in a multicentre, double-blind, controlled study on 1.072 elderly, to assess the resistance to respiratory infections. The product containing probiotics, well tolerated, induced a reduction in the duration of respiratory infections, especially URTI and nasopharyngitis.

10. Effects on digestive system [67]:

Many of the investigated effects of probiotics refer to the digestive system. These effects relate to both paraphysiological conditions, e.g. constipation and to situations of illness. A review has been published on the effect of probiotic strains on constipation: five clinical studies placebo-controlled were taken into consideration on a total of 377 subjects. The results show that favorable effects on stool frequency and stool consistency were obtained in adults with B. lactis DN-173 010, L. casei and E. coli Nissl 1917 probiotic strains. Some strains have led to a reduction in the perception of bloating (reported by patients before and after treatment). In children, the L. rhamnosus Lcr35 strain showed positive effects although not statistically significant (due to the low number of subjects involved) while the L. rhamnosus GG strain had no impact if compared to placebo.

11. Anti-diabetic activities of probiotics [71]:

According to the International Diabetes Federation (IDF) of Southeast Asia, 425 million people have diabetes worldwide including 78 million people in the Southeast Asian region. Based on large-scale 16 S rRNA gene sequencing, quantitative real-time PCR and fluorescent in situ hybridization, the connection between the composition of the intestinal microbiota and metabolic diseases, like obesity and diabetes, has been postulated by Larsen et al. Consequently, enhancing the benficial microbiota by the use of probiotics is expected to play a significant role in neutralization of the disorder.

Patients with type-2 diabetes have significantly reduced numbers of firmicutes species, such that the bacteroidetes/ firmicutes ratio has increased, which positively correlates with plasma glucose concentration. Management of type 2 diabetes by modulating gut hormones, such as gastric inhibitory polypeptide and glucagonlike peptide-1, via probiotic and prebiotic interventions is another convincing strategy. Currently, research is focused on generating new prebiotics, such as arabinoxylan and arabinoxylan oligosaccharides, which show promising results in counteracting related metabolic disorders, because both carbohydrates have been linked to adiposity reduction.

12. Anti-obesity activity of probiotics [71]:

Abnormal or excessive fat (obesity) accumulation that directly impairs health is linked to an increase in energy availability, sedentariness and a greater control of ambient temperature, leading to an imbalance in energy intake and expenditure.Probiotics possess physiological functions that contribute to the health of host environment regulating microbes. In most instances,weight loss is facilitated by thermogenic and lipolytic responses through stimulating the sympathetic nervous system. Probiotic strains, Lactobacillus gasseri BNR17 have shown properties of inhibiting the increase in adipocyte tissue that are the main source of leptin and adiponectin and thereby, limiting leptin secretion. Other probiotic microbes such as L. casei, Lactobacillus acidophilus and Bifidobacterium longum have also been reported to have hypocholesterolemic effects.

13. Anti-inflammatory activity of probiotics [71]

Crohn's disease (CD) and ulcerative colitis (UC) are among the most chronic inflammatory diseases of the GIT and are collectively called IBD.Research has shown that an imbalance in the gut microbiota plays an important pathophysiological role in the positive regulation of IBD. It is also understood that the disorder could possibly be altered by supplementation with probiotics, prebiotics, and synbiotics. IBD is being associated with impaired production of SCFAs, particularly, acetate, butyrate, and propionate. Moreover, these SCFAs have been known to play a key role in maintaining colonic homeostasis.Therefore, it is reasonable to consider that supplementation with indigestible carbohydrates and fiber (prebiotic) alone, or in combination with probiotics to increase the production of SCFAs could be useful therapeutic approaches.

Presently, progress in the field is mostly concerned with developing genetically engineered probiotic bacterial strains that are able to produce and discharge immunomodulators, such as interleukin-10, trefoil factors (compact proteins co-expressed with mucins in the GIT), or lipoteichoic acid (a major constituent of the cell wall of Gram-positive bacteria) that can impact the host immune system, resulting in the restoration of the level of protective commensal bacterial species.

14. Anti-cancer activity of probiotics [71]:

As per WHO cancer fact sheet, cancer has been a dreadful disease affecting peoples all over the globe. More than 70% of the global cancer deaths are from Asian, African, and American continents.Natural sources that confer anti-carcinogenic effects, such as probiotics have been receiving prime focus in recent years. These have attracted intense interest from clinical nutritionists, scientists, and industrialists to work in a collaborative manner to bring down the disease and develop an effective drug with minimal or no side-effects.

In vitro studies have demonstrated that probiotic strains, Lactobacillus fermentum NCIMB-5221 and -8829, have highly potent in suppressing colorectal cancer cells and promoting normal epithelial colon cell growth through the production of SCFAs (ferulic acid). This ability was also compared with other probiotics namely L. acidophilus ATCC 314 and L. rhamnosus ATCC 51303 both of which were previously characterized with tumorigenic activity.

Again two different probiotic strains L. acidophilus LA102 and L. casei LC232 have also been found to show pronounced cytotoxic activities, with in vitro anti-proliferative activity against two colorectal cancer cell lines (Caco-2 and HRT-18). Though probiotics could play a significant role in neutralizing cancer, research is limited only to in vitro tests.

15. Anti-allergic activity of probiotic:

The increasing prevalence of allergic diseases caused by immune disorders is a serious economic and social burden worldwide. Comprehending the fundamental molecular mechanism that contributes to the etiology of allergic diseases, as well as new treatment approaches is vital for the follow-up and prevention of these diseases [71]. Recent evidence suggests that exposure to bacteria in early life may exhibit a protective role against allergy and in this context probiotics may provide safe alternative microbial stimulation needed for the developing immune system in infants. In the same time they improve mucosal barrier function, a property that is considered to contribute in moderating allergic response [60].

A limited number of strains have been tested for their efficacy in the treatment and prevention of allergy in infants. In a recent study of breast fed infants suffering from atopic eczema B. lactis and L. rhamnosus GG were found to be effective in decreasing the eczema severity. Furthermore L. rhamnosus GG has been found successful in preventing the occurrence of atopic eczema in high risk infants, when supplied prenatally to selected mothers who had at least one first degree relative with atopic eczema, allergic rhinitis, or asthma [60].

In vitro studies of certain probiotics, such as Lactobacillus plantarum L67, have shown the potential to prevent allergy-associated disorders with the production of interleukin-12 and interferon-g in their host. In another study, L. plantarum 06CC2 significantly alleviated allergic symptoms and reduced the levels of total immunoglobulin E, ovalbumin-specifific immunoglobulin E, and histamine in the sera of ovalbumin-sensitized mice. In spleen cells of the mice, L. plantarum 06CC2 is known to significantly enhance the secretions of interferon-g and interleukin-4, which are responsible for alleviating allergic symptoms [71].

16. Angiogenic activity of probiotics [71]:

Angiogenesis has been an important phenomenon and is necessary for wound healing process through delineated cellular responses to regenerate damaged tissues.Deregulated angiogenesis has a prominent impact on major human diseases, such as cancer, diabetic retinopathy, and IBD including CD and UC. Non-pathogenic probiotic yeast, S. boulardii, has been reported to protect against intestinal injury and inflammation.The potential mechanisms of probiotics in angiogenesis process may include alteration of inflammatory cytokine profiles, down regulation of pro-inflammatory cascades or induction of regulatory mechanisms in a strain-specific manner, epithelial barrier function enhancement, visceral hypersensitivity reduction, spinal afferent traffic, and stress response.

17. Effect of probiotics on brain and CNS [71]:

The colonization of microbiota in the GIT is well-associated with both GIT and gastrointestinal diseases. Moreover, in recent years, many studies have been devoted towards elucidating the influence of gut microbiota on the CNS. The "microbiota-gut-brain axis" is an interactive, bi-directional communication established by the exchange of regulatory signals between the GIT and CNS. The effect of probiotics on the CNS has been mainly studied in clinical trials, where it has been evident that gut microbiota influence human brain development function. In children with autism spectrum disorder, a daily dose of L. plantarum WCFS1 (4.5 1010 CFU/ day) led to an improvement in their school records and attitude towards food.

Messaoudi et al discussed reduced psychological distress in a randomized trial involving healthy volunteers treated with oral administration of Lactobacillus helveticus R0052 and B. longum R0175. In another clinical trial, Rao et al showed a decrease in anxiety symptoms by administration of L. casei strain Shirota to patients suffering from chronic fatigue syndrome. Szajewska reported that autism spectrum and attention-deficit/ hyperactivity disorders in children could be prevented by L. rhamnosus administration to the mother at 4 weeks from expected delivery. It has been observed that many gut bacteria synthesize to neuroactive compounds similar to those produced in the host brain.

Human intestinally derived strains of L. brevis DPC6108 and Bifidobacterium dentium were reported to produce large amounts of g-aminobutyric acid, a brain neurotransmitter that helps humans to suppress anxiety and depression. Doses of a multispecies probiotic containing L. brevis W, B. lactis W, L. acidophilus W37, Bififidobacterium bififidum W2, L. salivarius W2, L. casei W5, and Lactococcus lactis (W19 and W58) to healthy humans showed a signifificant overall reduction in the cognitive reactivity to sad mood.Oral intake of L. acidophilus has been shown to assist people to regulate their mood towards rewards and addictive behavior.

18. Antibiotic-associated Diarrhoea [60]:

Mild or severe episodes of diarrhoea are common side effects of antibiotic therapy as the normal microflora tends to be suppressed, encouraging the overgrowth of opportunistic or pathogenic strains. Treatment consists of withdrawal of the causal antibiotic agent, correction of the electrolyte disorders, and in severe cases therapy with metronidazole or vancomycin. Treatment with probiotics has been used in clinical practice with L. rhamnosus and S. boulardii being administered. Several studies that have been carried out suggest that probiotic use is associated with a reduced risk of antibiotic-associated diarrhoea. A meta-analysis evaluating the available evidence on probiotics for the prevention and treatment of antibiotic-associated diarrhoea concluded that probiotic administration- (namely, L. rhamnosus, L. casei, and the yeast S. boulardii, as these are the probiotics predominantly included in the majority of trials) is associated with a reduced risk of the condition.

19. Probiotic use in infectious diarrhoea [60]:

Treatment and prevention of infectious diarrhoea are probably the most widely accepted health benefits of probiotic microorganisms. Rotavirus is the most common cause of acute infantile diarrhoea in the world and a significant cause of infant mortality.Probiotic supplementation of infant formulas has been aimed both at the prevention of rotaviral infections and the treatment of established disease. Well-controlled clinical studies have shown that probiotics such as L. rhamnosus GG, L. reuteri, L. casei Shirota, and B. animalis Bb12 can shorten the duration of acute rotavirus diarrhoea with the strongest evidence pointing to the effectiveness of L. rhamnosus GG and B. animalis Bb12. The proposed mechanisms include competitive blockage of receptor site signals regulating secretory and motility defences, enhancement of the immune response, and production of substances that directly inactivate the viral particles.

In a prospective, randomized, controlled French study conducted among children in day care, the administered probiotic yoghurt product containing L. casei shortened the mean duration of diarrhoea significantly compared to the conventional one. Several studies have investigated the efficacy of probiotics in the prevention of travellers' diarrhoea in adults. Although results are quite contradictory, due to differences in study populations, type of probiotic being investigated, applied doses, as well as trip destination and traveller compliance, L.rhamnosus GG, S. boulardii, L. acidophilus, and B. bifidum seem to exhibit significant efficacy.

20. Radiation induced diarrhoea [65]:

A double blind, placebo controlled trial was done to investigate the efficacy of a high potency probiotic preparation on prevention of radiation – induced diarrhoea in cancer patients. About 490 patients, who underwent adjuvant postoperative radiation therapy, were given either high potency probiotic preparation VSL#3 or placebo. Efficacy end points were incidence and severity of radiation-induced diarrhoea and daily number of bowel movements. Results were- more placebo patients had radiation induced diarrhoea than VSL #3 patients and more patients given placebo suffered grade 3 or 4 diarrhoea compared with VSL #3 recipients. So it was concluded that probiotic lactic acid producing bacteria are an easy, safe and feasible approach to protect cancer patients against the risk of radiation.

21. Constipation [61]:

Constipation is a major digestive complaint among the elderly, in particular the institutionalised. Although also, otherwise healthy, adults and hospitalised subjects may experience constipation. Constipated subjects have been observed to have a modified faecal micro flora with reduced levels of bifidobacteria, Bacteroides and, in particular, reduced levels of clostridia. Probiotics have been suggested to relieve constipation. However, review of the literature does not substantiate this claim. This may relate to the causes of constipation; physical inactivity, low-fibre diets, insufficient liquid intake and some drugs. The altered microflora composition is more likely to be a consequence than the cause of constipation, correcting the micro flora composition may therefore not be of help.

22. Traveller's diarrhoea [92]:

Traveler's diarrhoea is a common health complaint among travelers. Rates of traveler's diarrhoea can range from five to 50% depending upon destination. A meta-analysis was done on published randomized controlled clinical trials of traveler's diarrhoea cases. It was concluded that probiotics significantly prevent traveler's diarrhoea. Saccharomyces boulardii and a mixture of Lactobacillus acidophilus and Bifidobacterium bifidum had significant efficacy.

23. Helicobacter pylori [65]:

H. pylori, is a major cause of chronic gastritis and peptic ulcer and a risk factor for gastric malignancies. Antibiotics based H. pylori eradication treatment is 90% effective. However, it is expensive and causes side effects and antibiotic resistance. Various studies revealed that Probiotics had an in vitro inhibitory effect, reduced H. pylori associated gastric inflammation in animals, improved H. pylori associated gastritis and also probiotic treatment reduced H. pylori therapy associated side effects.

24. Inflammatory bowel disease [65]:

Inflammatory bowel disease classically includes ulcerative colitis and Crohn's disease representing different patterns of chronic inflammation of GIT. Recent clinical and experimental observation implicates an imbalance in the intestinal mucosa with relative predominance of aggressive bacteria and relative paucity of protective bacteria and also stimulation of pro-inflammatory immunological mechanisms. Various preliminaries studies suggest a positive response to probiotics in patients with IBD, causing decreased expression of inflammatory markers ex-vivo, increasing the immune response and improving the gut barrier functions. Thus, probiotics have a potential for inducing or maintaining remissions in IBD. However, further studies are required to have a proven beneficial role in IBD cases. Limited data from small controlled studies would suggest that VSL#3 is a reasonable therapy in the primary and secondary type of pouchitis

A. Ulcerative colitis: (UC)[93]:

UC like IBD mainly affects the lining of the large intestine and rectum. Long-standing UC is a risk factor for colon cancer. Use of various probiotic species like S. boulardii, Lactobacillus casei and Bifidobacterium bifidum has shown promising results. A pilot study suggested that fermented milk containing B. breve, B. bifidum and L. acidophilus was beneficial to induce mild degree remission in patients.

B. Crohn's disease: (CD) [93]:

Crohn's disease is a form of IBD which usually affects the intestine, but may occur anywhere from the mouth to the end of the rectum. CD causes ulceration and inflammation that affects the body's ability to digest food, absorb nutrients and eliminate waste in a healthy way. Salmonella, Campylobacter jejuni, Clostridium difficile, Adenovirus, and Mycoplasma have been identified as some of the common causative agents.The therapeutic effects of probiotic consumption on CD are reported to be due to competitive action with commensal, pathogenic flora and an influence on the immune response system. Probiotics also prevent IBD by restoring integrity of the protective intestinal mucosa.

C. Pouchitis [93]

Pouchitis is another type of IBD where ileal pouch gets inflamed especially after colectomy and ileal pouch canal anastomosis. In different studies the VSL#3 pro biotic mixture was found to be highly effective for maintain ing remission of chronic pouchitis. Probiotics may also influence the mucosal cell-cell interactions and cellular stability by enhancement of intestinal barrier function by modulating cytoskeletal and tight junctional protein phosphorylation, and also by producing anti-oxidant enzymes such as superoxide dismutase and catalase thus ameliorating the IBD symptoms.

25. Surgical infections [65]:

Before the advent of antiseptics and antibiotics, fermented milk was used for healing wounds and to fight infections. Recent studies show some success in application of probiotics for treating and preventing surgical infections. Studies shows L.fermentum RC-14 was shown to significantly inhibit S. aureus infection and bacterial adherence to surgical implants also.[50] L. plantarum 299 with oat fibres for one week had significantly fewer episodes of infection and pancreatic abscesses. Also, these studies indicate the role of probiotics to decontaminate the intestine prior to gut surgery instead of antibiotics.

26. Probiotic use in Lactose intolerance [60]:

Lactose intolerance is a genetically determined beta-galactosidase deficiency resulting in the inability to hydrolyse lactose into the monosaccharides glucose and galactose. Upon reaching the large bowel the undigested lactose is degraded by bacterial enzymes leading to osmotic diarrhoea. Lactose intolerant individuals develop diarrhoea, abdominal discomfort, and flatulence after consumption of milk or milk products. Although conventional yoghurt preparations, using S. thermophilus and L. delbrueckii ssp. Bulgaricus, are even more effective in this direction, partly because of higher betagalactosidase activity, improvement of lactose metabolism is a claimed health benefit attributed to probiotics and seems to involve certain strains more than others and in specific concentrations.

27. Probiotics and calcium absorption [103]:

Milk is considered to be abundant with calcium apart from other dietary sources. Individuals with lactose intolerance may probably develop osteoporosis due to decreased consumption of milk containing diet. Calcium absorption is favored in acidic pH. So if probiotics are fed to lactose intolerance patients, then milk lactose is hydrolyzed by probiotic strains, favoring calcium absorption.

28. Probiotic effectiveness in Necrotising Enterocolitis [65]:

(NE) – NE is one devastating intestinal disorder that a preterm infant may face in a neonatal intensive care unit (NICU). It is characterized by abdominal distension, bilious vomiting, bloody diarrhoea, lethargy, apnoea, and bradycardia. NE is reported in 10 to 25% of preterm infants, admitted to NICU and may affect 1/3 to1/2 of all low birth weight infants. The mortality ranges from 20 to 30% and those who survive have long term sequalae as short gut syndrome, intestinal obstruction and multi-organ failure. Low birth weight pre-term infant delivered by Caesarean section often require intensive care and are breast fed only after several days. The normal process by which organisms such as lactobacillus species are ingested via vaginal birth and propagated by mother's milk does not take place in these infants. Therefore these infants are exposed to a plethora of pathogenic microbes like – Clostridium, Escherichia, Salmonella, Shigella, Campylobacter, Pseudomonas, Streptococcus, Enterococcus, Staphylococcus and coagulase negative Staphylococcus, which colonize the intestine and increase the risk of NE..Further, pre-term infants, given formula feeding have less Lactobacillus and Bifidobacterium species in their stool compared to controls. These findings suggest a correlation between NE and Lactobacillus species.

A human trial with 2.5 x 108 live Lactobacillus acidophilus and 2.5 x 108 live Bifidobacterium infantis given to 1237 newborn in Columbia, resulted in 60% reduction in NE and overall mortality. A correlation between normal gut microflora and protection against various infections has been reported. This supports the concept of early intestinal colonization with organisms such as Lactobacillus rhamnosus and Bifidobacterium infantis and subsequent protection against NE.

29. Probiotics in critical illness [65]:

Some studies propose that probiotics have an important emerging role in managing critical illnesses originating in gastrointestinal tract like acute pancreatitis. In cirrhotic patients, probiotics have shown a decrease in incidence of encephalopathy. Also reduction of post liver transplant infective complication using probiotics have been seen.It also helps in colonic involvement in Stevens –Johnson syndrome. Probiotic Lactobacillus reuteri reduces gingivitis and decreases gum bleeding.

30. Probiotics in veterinary practice [103]:

They are marketed as either pastes or powders and are commonly given to young foals, horses being trailered or in competition. These products are commonly defined as live microbial feed supplements.

31. Acute otitis media [94]:

Acute otitis media is a common viral infection which becomes infected by bacteria in young children and is characterized by acute ear pain . Children with acute otitis media have been observed to harbour fewer α-hemolytic Streptococci in the nasopharynx than those resistant to acute otitis media.

After spraying α -hemolytic Stretococci into the nose of 108 otitis-prone children regularly for 10 days and the final administration of the 'booster dose' after 2 months, 42% (22 of 53) of the children in the placebo group remained healthy during follow-up period and had a normal tympanic membrane as compared with 22% (12 of 55) of the children in the placebo group. The spray was administered immediately after the antibiotic therapy and consisted of two Streptococcus sanguinis strains, two Streptococcus mitis strains and one Streptococcus oralis strain, in equal proportions.

Hatakka and coworkers examined the effect of probiotic capsules containing two L. rhamnosus strains, one Bifidobacterium breve strain, one Propionibacterium freudenreichii strains in otitis prone children. The probiotic treatment showed the tendency to decrease but not significantly reduce the occurrence of acute otitis media.

Probiotic milk containing L. rhamnosus GG promoted the nasal colonization of Staphylococcus aureus, Streptococcus pneumoniae and β-hemolytic Streptococci and had initial effects on respiratory tract infections in children attending day care centers.

32. Voice prostheses [94]:

A voice prosthesis is an artificial device, usually made up of silicone that is used to help the laryngectomized patients to speak. This device has a very short life time because of the excessive growth of the microorganisms, especially Candida species on its surface. As a result, there is improper closure of the valve of prostheses leading to leakage of food into the wind pipe, causing breathing troubles. Since yeast and bacterial colonization of esophageal side of prosthesis impedes fluent speech, respiration and swallowing because of either leakage or increased airflow resistance. Therefore, it is needed to replace the voice prostheses regularly, every 1-2 weeks to 3-4 months.

In a study, the buttermilk containing Lactobacillus lactis and Lactococcus lactis ssp. cremoris and a fermented milk drink containing L. casei Shirota were examined for their ability to decrease the amount of bacteria and yeast on voice prostheses in both in vitro and in vivo studies. The results showed that the consumption of fermented milk containing L. casei Shirota increased the lifetime of voice prostheses by four times.

33. Application of Probiotics in Animal Feed and Aquaculture [4]:

Animal feed companies and researchers have been looking for alternative products and strategies that can help to maintain animal gut health in order to prevent or reduce the prevalence of pathogens in the food chain. An alternative and effective approach to antibiotic administration to livestock is the use of probiotics, which can help to improve gut microbial balance and therefore the natural defence of the animal against pathogenic bacteria.The use of probiotics and commercial products containing probiotics in aquaculture (e.g.

shrimp production) has shown similar results compared to the antimicrobials currently used. It could be an interesting alternative to overcome the problem of antibiotic resistance.

Multiple ways exist in which probiotics could be beneficial and these could act either singly or in combination forming a single probiotic. These include:

(i) inhibition of a pathogen via production of antagonistic compounds,

(ii) competition for attachment sites,

(iii) competition for nutrients,

(iv) alteration of enzymatic activity of pathogens,

(v) immunostimulatory functions and

(vi) nutritional benefits such as improving feed digestibility and feed utilization.

Verschuere et al suggested a new definition of a probiotic for aquatic environments: 'a live microbial adjunct which has a beneficial effect on the host by modifying the host-associated or ambient microbial community, by ensuring improved use of the feed or enhancing its nutritional value, by enhancing the host's response towards disease, or by improving the quality of its ambient environment', or that 'a probiotic is an entire microorganism or its components that are beneficial to the health of the host'.

Probiotic strain	Application	Probiotic effect
Bacillus subtilis, Bacilluslicheniformis	shrimp production	reduce stress, improve health, the quality of water, clean effluent water, control pathogenic bacteria and their virulence, stimulate the immune system, improve gut flora, substitute antibiotics, improve growth
Bacillus spp. and yeasts	mollusc production	minimize diseases caused by Vibrio spp. and Aeromonas spp., which results in mollusc mortality
Clostridium spp.	freshwater fish feed	produces digestive enzymes, which facilitate feed utilization and digestion, antibacterial activity against pathogenic

		microorganisms
Bacillus spp., Saccharomyces cerevisiae	aquaculture	improve water quality and interaction with phytoplankton, possess adhesion abilities, produce bacteriocins, provide immunostimulation
Bacillus spp., S. cerevisiae	aquaculture	stimulate the growth of microalgae that produce organic extracts capable of inhibiting pathogens and vibrios, then some microalgae species produce the antibiotic thiotropocin against some pathogens
S. cerevisiae	aquaculture	immunostimulatory activity, produces inhibitory substances against pathogens
Bifidobacterium longum, L. plantarum	chicken feed	produce antimicrobial substances against pathogens such as Campylobacter
Pediococcus acidilactici, Lactococcus lactis, L. casei, Enterococcus faecium	weaned piglet	stimulate animal growth, reduce coliform counts by the production of antimicrobial metabolites
S. cerevisiae	Lactating ruminants	facilitates increased mobilization of body reserves, increases milk fatty acid production
S. cerevisiae	Camel feed	increases total mass gain and improves feed utilization
S. cerevisiae	Buffalo feed	increases digestion of cellulose
Pediococcus acidilactici	broiler chickens	improves performance, reduces serum cholesterol
Lactobacillus, Bifidobacterium, Streptococcus, Enterococcus ssp.	layer hens	reduces mortality
L. sporogenes	broiler chickens	reduces serum total cholesterol and triglycerides

Lactobacillus ssp.	chicken feed	immunomodulating properties
Lactobacillus spp., Bacillus spp.	poultry feed	reduces zoonosis in poultry meat
L. reuteri LPB P01-001	swine feed	mass gain, antimicrobial activity against E. coli and S. aureus
Enterococcus faecalis, E. faecium	canine feed	bacteriocin-like inhibitory substances, antimicrobial activity against Gram(+) bacteria, colonize transiently

Table 7: Application and effects of probiotics in animal feed and aquaculture [4]

34. PROBIOTICS AND COVID-19

In December 2019 a viral outbreak referred to as COVID-19 has been reported from Wuhan, China. The viral agent has been recognised as a zoonotic beta-coronavirus, named severe acute respiratory syndrome coronavirus 2 (SARS-CoV-2), similar to other SARS and MERS (Middle East Respiratory Syndrome) coronaviruses . COVID-19 causes a severe acute respiratory syndrome (SARS) named specifically SARS-CoV-2 [117].

Post-mortem analysis on a patient died by SARS-CoV-2 conducted by these authors on lung, liver and hearth tissue that had shown severe damages at lungs with oedema and desquamation, evident symptoms of breath complications and fatigue. Some patients with COVID-19 showed intestinal microbial dysbiosis with decreased probiotics such as Lactobacillus and Bifidobacterium, suggesting the needing to assess nutritional and gastrointestinal function for all patients [118] .

Nutritional support and application of prebiotics or probiotics were suggested also in COVID-19 infected patients, to regulate the balance of intestinal microbiota and reduce the risk of secondary infection due to bacterial translocation. Other authors have speculated that COVID-19 may be related to the gut microbiota, since some evidence highlighted a secondary gut infection or disfunction in patient with RTIs, probably due also to antibiotics which are not selective towards harmful bacteria. This suggest also a gut–lung crosstalk, and in some extent that the symptoms may be modulated by probiotics, altering in this way the gastrointestinal symptoms favourably and protecting also the respiratory system [119].

Probiotic as antiviral agents:

The human respiratory tract is exposed to several microorganisms. It is the primary path for the internalization of respiratory viruses. Thus, preventing the virus's adsorption onto the mucosal epithelial surfaces is crucial for reducing disease development. The human body harbors a range of mutually beneficial microorganisms. Collectively, we denote them as the human microbiota. Probiotics are also one such friendly set of microbes that positively influence human health when ingested or administered in a particular concentration. Probiotic strains of Lactobacillus and Bifidobacterium genera can trap the virus and interfere in the virus binding to the host cell recep tors, which is beneficial to the host health. Similarly, probiotics administration confers health benefits to humans against respiratory viral infections, including Respiratory syncytial virus and Influenza A virus (IFV) [120].

GUT-LUNG AXIS and COVID-19

The gastrointestinal tract and lung are among the body compartments that host microbiota; however, the lung has a small number of microbiota when compared to that of the gut. There is accumulating evidence that bidirectional communications exist between gut and lung, which is called the gut-lung axis. This bidirectional crosstalk is involved in the support of immune homeostasis. It is believed that the gastrointestinal inflammation results in lung inflammation through this connection. It has been shown previously that dysbiosis of gut microbiota is linked with several respiratory pathological conditions and shifts in the composition of the lung microbiota toward the gut microbiota have been observed in several respiratory disorders. One of the suggested mechanisms behind the bidirectional interaction between lung and gut microbiota systems is that increased permeability of the GI tract allows the leakage and migration of the gut microbiota to the lung, modulating its microbiota and thus its immune responses. It was found that

COVID-19 patients with GI symptoms such as diarrhea experienced more severe respiratory disorders than those without GI symptoms [121].

Probiotic effects on immune responses:

Boosting immune responses during the incubation and non-severe stages of Covid-19 infection, to eliminate the virus and preclude disease progression to severe stages, have been proposed as extremely important. In the gastrointestinal tract (GIT), known as one of the most microbiologically active ecosystems playing a crucial role in the working of the mucosal immune system, probiotics stimulate the immune system and induce a network of signals mediated by the whole bacteria or their cell wall structure. Many probiotic effects are mediated through immune regulation, particularly through balance control of proinflammatory and anti-inflammatory cytokines. Another important effect exerted by probiotics is to enforce and maintain the integrity of junction between enterocytes, in this way entrance of SARSCoV2 is reduced, as well as the risk to develop COVID-19 [119].

Putative mechanisms by which probiotics may help manage coronavirus infection [120]

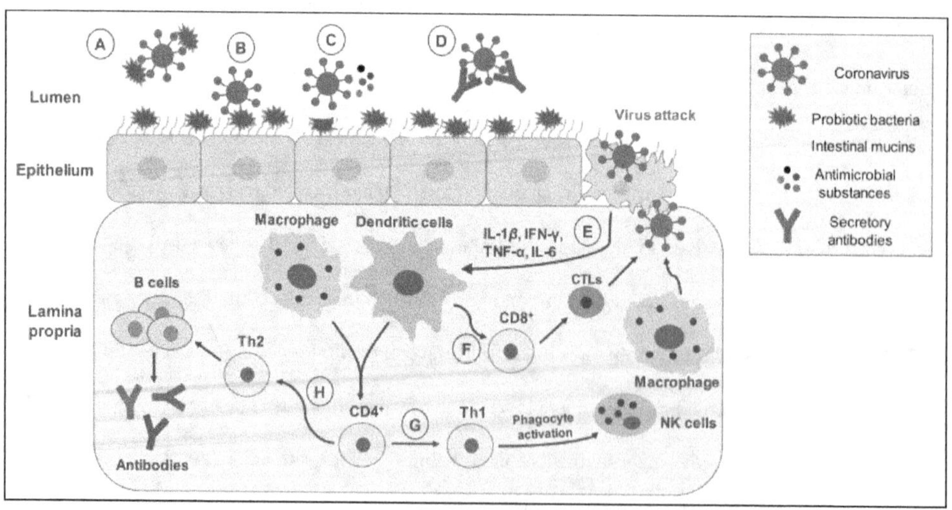

Figure 7: Management of Coronavirus by Probiotics

(**A**) Probiotic bacteria can hinder the adsorption process via directly binding to the virus and inhibiting entry into epithelial cells.

(**B**) Binding of probiotic bacteria to the epithelial surface can cause steric hindrance and block the virus's attachment to the host cell receptor.

(**C**) Probiotic bacteria releases antimicrobial substances (such as bacteriocins, biosurfactants, lactic acid, hydrogen peroxide, nitric oxide, organic acids) and intestinal mucins from mucosal cells, which can effectively inhibit virus proliferation.

(**D**) Virus neutralized by secretory antibodies like IgA.

(**E**) Upon virus attack in epithelial cells, probiotics mediate their antiviral effects by eliciting immune responses by activating macrophages and dendritic cells.

(**F**) Activation of immune response leads to differentiating CD8+ T lymphocytes into CTLs, capable of destroying virus-infected cells.

(**G**) CD4+ T lymphocytes cells differentiate into Th1, which activates phagocytosis through NK cells and macrophages, promoting pathogen killing.

(**H**) CD4+ cells differentiate into Th2 cells, which induce B-cells' proliferation that produces antibodies like IgA, IgG, and IgM. CTLs, cytotoxic T-lymphocytes; Th1, T-helper cells type 1.

Probiotics and Prebiotics: ACE inhibitory effect:

The directly or indirectly positive impact of probiotics on the ACE enzymes is well stated. During food fermentation, probiotics produce bioactive peptides with the capability to inhibit the ACE enzymes by blocking the active sites. Moreover, the debris of the dead probiotic cells acted also as ACE inhibitors. These findings suggest that probiotics could be a potential blocker to the ACE receptor that acts as a gateway for SARS-CoV-2 to attack GI cells. The concept of using drugs to block the ACE receptors as a treatment approach against COVID-19 was proposed by Fernández-Fernández, despite the otherwise opinion expressed by Esler and Esler. Imai et al have stated a positive inflfluence of using an ACE blocker to reduce respiratory distress syndrome.

Prebiotics may also have an excellent potential effect against COVID-19 by enhancing probiotics growth and survivability. Furthermore, prebiotics could have a direct effect on GI symptoms caused by COVID-19 via blocking the ACE enzymes.

Some patients with COVID-19 exhibited intestinal microbial dysbiosis characterized by low numbers of different probiotic species such as Bifidobacterium and Lactobacillus. This is could be an indicator of their weak immunity, and therefore, it has been suggested that these patients require nutritional support and prebiotic or probiotic supplementation to re-normalize the intestinal flora balance and decrease the risk of infection [121].

Possible application of probiotics in reducing burden and severity of Sars-CoV-2 infections [123]

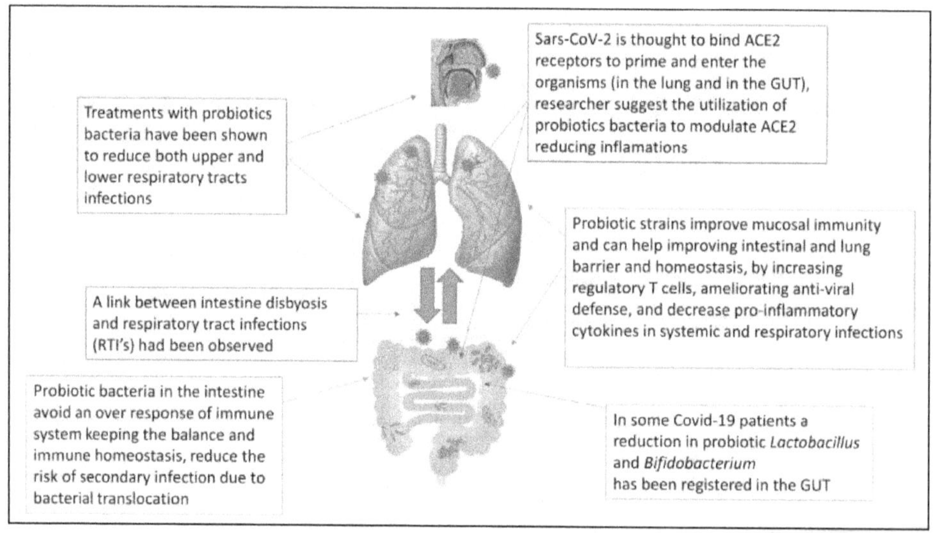

Figure 8: Probiotics in reducing burden and severity of Sars-CoV-2 infections

Preclinical studies on mice (A) and clinical studies in humans (B) in COVID-19 infection management [124].

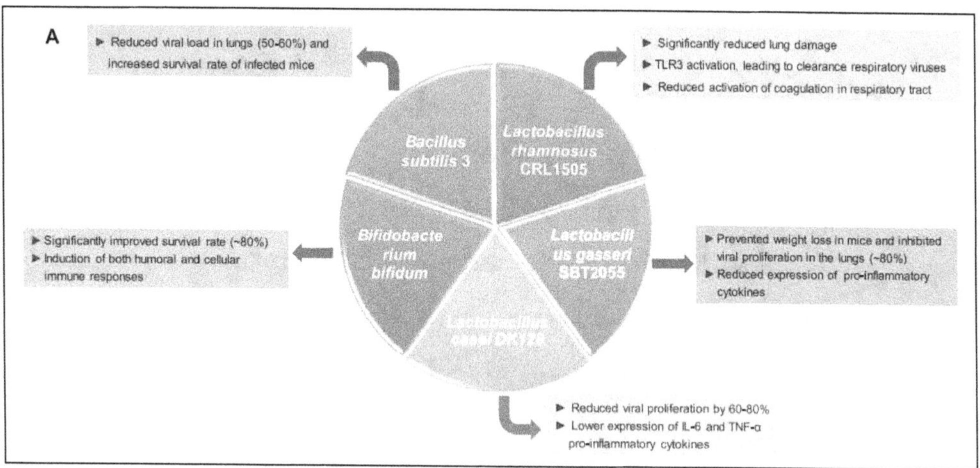

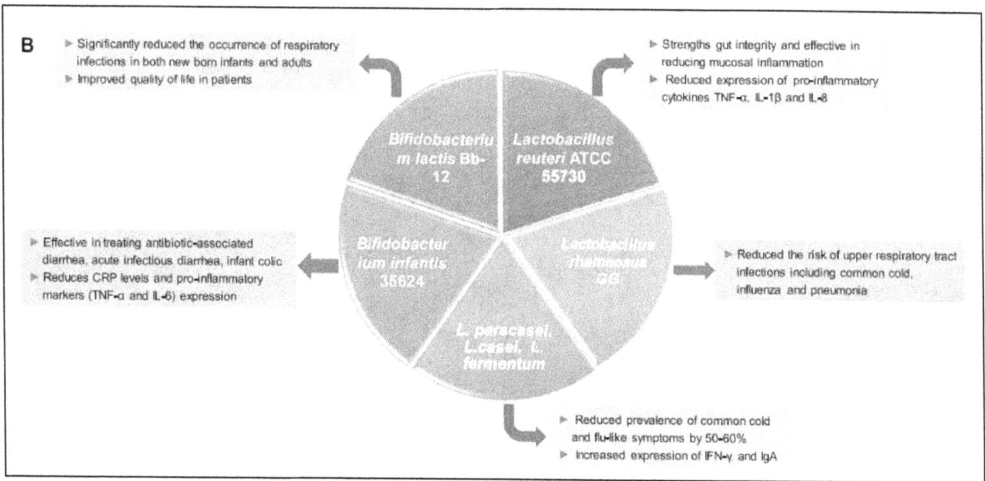

Figure 9: Preclinical and clinical studies in COVID-19 infection management

PROBIOTICS: THE PAST, PRESENT AND FUTURE

Past: Probiotics were originally used to influence both animal and human health through intestinal microbiota alterations.

Present: Specific live microbial food ingredients and their effects on human health are studied both within food matrices and as single or mixed culture preparations. It has been proposed that inactivated microbes and their components can also have probiotic effects.The probiotic potential of different bacterial strains, even within the same species, differs; different strains of the same species are always unique, and may have differing areas of adherence (site-specific), specific immunological effects, and actions on a healthy versus an inflamed mucosal milieu may be distinct from each other.

Future: Probiotic research should aim at characterization of the healthy normal gut microbiota in each individual, assessing the species composition as well as concentrations of different bacteria in each part of the intestine[7].

DEVELOPING FUTURE PROBIOTIC STRAINS

Quality of probiotic strains

Probiotics are special ingredients that are used in both foods and pharmaceutical or special dietary applications. They have been selected to express strain specific properties which are important for their proposed health effects. Such characteristics should be retained through food and pharmaceutical processes and storage to be of benefit to the consumer. The most important factor is to retain the strain characteristics and the purity of the preparation. It has been reported that especially dried probiotic preparations may have contaminants. This sets the requirements for hygienic preparation of the products and careful identification of the strains used.

Unlike pharmaceuticals or food chemicals such as additives, the quality criteria for probiotics are largely undefined. This is a key factor for health effects as long term transfer of probiotic lactic acid bacteria or bifidobacteria in food processing along with the storage may result in changes in their characteristics and health properties [104].

Non-viable probiotics

Most definitions of probiotic bacteria stress the importance of the viability of the microbes. However, very little research has been done on non-viable probiotics. Non-viable probiotics would have several advantages over viable ones: longer shelf life, improved safety and no need for refrigerated storage or transport. Review of the literature suggests that non-viable probiotics may have positive health effects as well. This has been shown for shortening of rotavirus diarrhoea and alleviation of lactose intolerance [104].

LIMITATIONS

Our understanding of mechanisms involved in beneficial effects of probiotics, probiotics as well as synbiotics is rather superficial [93].Probiotics are regulated as dietary supplements and not subjected to the same rigorous standards as medications. A challenge with these products involves the complexity of quality control with live microorganisms. As a result, individuals may obtain a product that is ineffective or that contains varying quantities of bacteria or yeast. Published studies involving probiotics have often utilized small sample sizes and lacked appropriate randomization, blinding, or control groups. Therefore, the results from many probiotic studies should be interpreted cautiously due to methodological limitations. There is also heterogeneity among studies, since different probiotic doses, strains, treatment durations, and patient populations may have been used. Since probiotic effects are specific to a particular strain, this may have important implications when interpreting meta-analyses, particularly if strain designations were not provided [66].

CONCLUSION

Correction of the properties of unbalanced indigenous microbiota forms the rationale of probiotic therapy [7]. There is scientific evidence supporting the incorporation of probiotics in nutrition as a means of derivation of health benefits. Probiotics possess important functional attributes that could fulfill most of our basic nutritional and clinical supplementation requirements. Probiotics have demonstrated efficacy in preventing and treating various medical conditions, particularly those involving the gastrointestinal tract. Data supporting their role in other conditions are often conflicting. The best documented effects include bowel disorders such as lactose intolerance, antibiotic-associated diarrhoea and infectious diarrhoea associated with rotavirus, IBS and food allergies. Moreover, the contribution of probiotics in preventing and treatment of diabetes, obesity, cancer and diseases related to pathogenic microbes is an exciting and rapidly advancing research arena. [71]. Dairy products, particularly yoghurt, continue to be the most important vehicles for delivery of probiotic bacteria to the consumer with the nondairy sector continuously evolving as well, as a result of food technology advances and the growing demand [60]. With this knowledge, optimal probiotic strains can be developed. The viability of probiotics is a key parameter for developing probiotic food products. New technologies have been developed to enable high cell yield at large scale and ensure probiotic stability for a long period in food[4]. Nevertheless, the development of probiotics for human consumption is still in its infancy. Further research, in the form of controlled human studies, is needed to determine which probiotics and which dosages are associated with the greatest efficacy and for which patients, as well as to demonstrate their safety and limitations. In addition, the regulatory status of probiotics as food components needs to be established on an international level with emphasis on efficacy, safety, and validation of health claims on food labels. Introduction of antibiotic revolutionized the field of medicines. After introduction of antibiotics life expectancy increased. And it greatly improved the quality of human life by decreasing the mortality rate throughout the world [103].

Respiratory viral infections are one of the fastest escalating global disease burdens with high mortality rates. The disease severity can range from mild upper tract airway infection to severe chronic inflammation of the mucosal layer in the respiratory tract and multi-organ failure in some patients. At this point, the SARS-CoV-2 pandemic has caused severe mortality in several countries, and yet no precise drug regimen is available to the world population. Improving/strengthening human host immunity is one of the best prophylactic approaches to reduce the severity of such viral diseases [103].

On the basis of the available evidence, the possible benefits of probiotic administration in the framework of Covid-19 infection, may be due, principally, to their effects on innate and adaptive immunity. Probiotic actions such as influence on cytokines production by intestinal epithelial cells, IgA secretion stimulation to improve mucosal immunity, activation of phagocytosis and macrophage production, modulation of levels and function of regulatory cells, and induction of dendritic cells maturation, likely affect systemic inflammation. Furthermore, increasing evidence supports a link between the gut and lungs, thus, further studies should be addressed to investigate a potential role of probiotic in attenuating Covid-19 either through immunomodulatory actions on systemic inflammation or by direct interaction with the lungs [119].

It is evident that probiotics can reduce the incidence and severity of diseases, suggesting their promise for treating or preventing COVID-19. Probiotics could help prevent COVID-19 by maintaining the human GI or lung microbiota because dysbiosis plays a major role in the susceptibility of people to infectious diseases. In vitro and clinical studies are required to examine the potential preventive and curative effects of probiotics against SARS-CoV-2 infection. [121].

PART II

PROBIOTICS AND ORAL HEALTH

INTRODUCTION

Oral health is a vital component of health. World Health Organization defines it as a state of being free from chronic mouth and facial pain, oral and throat cancer, oral sores, birth defects such as cleft lip and palate, periodontal (gum) disease, tooth decay and tooth loss, and other diseases and disorders that affect the oral cavity. Global health preventive programs adopted worldwide have substantially contributed to reducing the extent and the severity of common oral diseases. Yet the prevalence of periodontal diseases and caries, both having microbial components in their etiology, remain high. Caries affects practically everyone in the global population at some stages of life while 15 – 35% of the adult population in industrialized countries is estimated to have periodontitis [105].

ORAL MICROBIOTA

There are around 1,000 species found in the human subgingival plaque and in the dorsum of the tongue. Among those, Lactobacilli make approximately 1% of the detected oral microflora whereas the whole microbiota is present in planktonic state or is finely integrated in oral biofilm on various oral surfaces. All different species coexist and interact within the biofilm which dynamically changes in complexity and amount; moreover, species depend on each other on survival [106].

Genera	Strain
Streptococcus	S. mutans, S. sanguis, S. anginosus, S. inter medius
Actinomyces/Aggregatibacter	Aggregatibacter actinomycetemcomitans, Actinomyces viscosus
Veillonella	V. parvula
Fusobacterium	F. nucleatum
Porphyromonas	P. gingivalis
Treponema	T. denticola
Bacteroides	Porphyromonas gingivalis, Prevotella intermedia/nigrescens, Tannerella forsythia
Campylobacter	C. Rectus
Eubacterium	E. nodatum, E. brachy, E. timidum
LactobacilluS	L. plantarum L. casei/paracasei, L. fermentum, L. acidophilus, L. salivarius, L. gasseri
Bifidobacterium	C. bifidus, B. dentium, B. longum, Scardovia nopinata, Parascardovia denticolens, Alloscardovia omnicolens
Capnocytophaga	C. gingivalis, C. ochracea
Peptostreptococcus	P. micros

| Staphylococcus | S. aureus |
| Selenomonas | S. noxia |

Table 8: Organisms found in oral cavity[107]

ORAL IMMUNOSYSTEM

Lactobacilli seems to play an important role in the microecological balance in the oral cavity where the oral tolerance is finely tuned by mucosal surfaces which represent a major site of pathogen entry, and the immune system is able to mount an effective response to protect the body from invading microorganisms, while maintaining tolerance to "harmless" antigens.

The oral cavity behaving as a gateway, to the underlying gastrointestinal tract, is the first site of contact between probiotics and the host. Despite structural similarities with other parts of the digestive system, oral cavity is unique for its highly specialized functions and characteristic site-specific pathology. Immunity in the oral cavity is mediated by the presence of diffuse lymphoid aggregates within the Waldeyer's ring and lymphatic tissues within lingual, pharyngeal tonsils and adenoids. Dendritic Langherans cells, located intraepithelially, process the oral antigen in the MHC-II cellular compartment and migrate to the closest regional lymph node to prime naïve T cells. Oral epithelial cells produce a range of cytokines as interleukin-1beta (IL-1beta), interleukin-6 (IL-6), tumor necrosis factor alfa (TNF-alfa), granulocyte macrophage colony stimulating factor (GM-CSF),transforming growth factor- beta (TGF-beta) and their receptors and interleukin-8 (IL-8) [108]. Microbial products play a key role in dendritic cell (DC) response through the pattern recognition receptors, which include Toll like receptors (TLR). Signals from DC can determine whether tolerance or an active immune response occurs to a particular antigen and furthermore, influence whether a Th1 or Th2 immune response predominates [109].

PROBIOTIC STRAINS IN THE ORAL CAVITY [110]

1. S. Salivarius

2. L. rhamnosus GG

3. L. acidophilus

4. L. casei

5. L. reuteri

6. Bififidobacterium DN-173 010

7. Propionibacterium freudenreichii ssp.

8. L. rhamnosus

9. L. paracasei

10. L. johnsonii

11. W. cibaria

12. L. casei Shirota

POTENTIAL MECHANISMS OF PROBIOTIC EFFECTS IN THE ORAL CAVITY

The general mechanisms of probiotics can be divided into three main categories:

(i) normalization of the intestinal microbiota,

(ii) modulation of the immune response, and

(iii) metabolic effects [112]

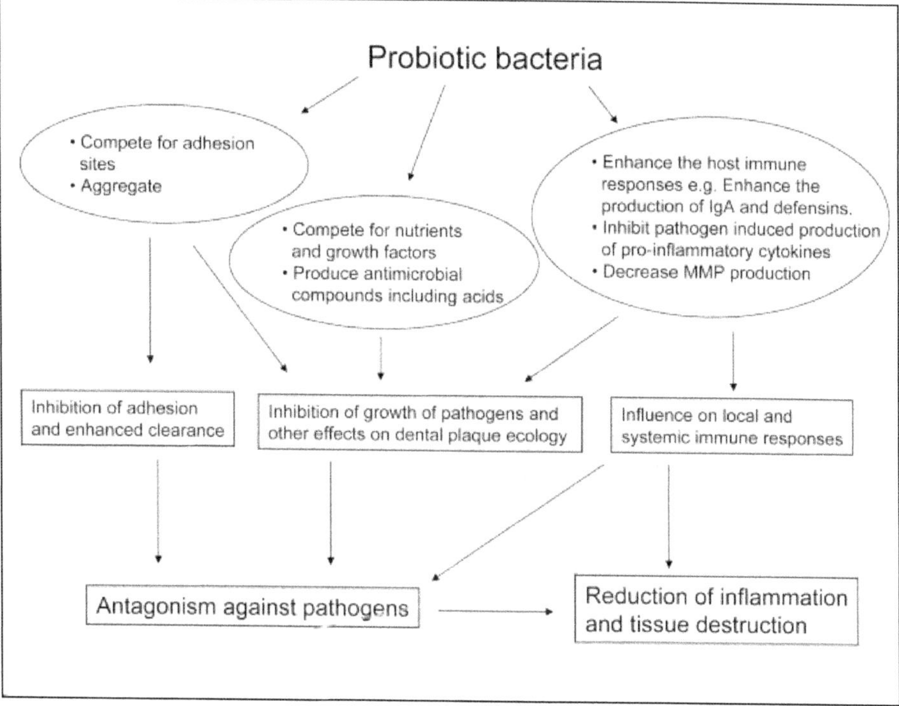

Figure 6: Mechanisms by which probiotic bacteria affect oral health [112]

The Probiotics have a three step action mechanism [94] -

i. Stimulates and modulates immune response,

ii. Normalize intestinal microflora

➢ ☐ Ensures colonization resistance

› □   Controls irritable bowel syndrome and other inflammatory bowel diseases.

iii. And also have the metabolic effects like- □

›   Bile salt deconjugation and secretion,

› □   Lactose hydrolysis,

› □   Reduction in toxigenic and mutagenic reactions in gut. □

›   Supply of nutrients to colon epithelium.

ORIGIN AND VEHICLES FOR PROBIOTIC DELIVERY

Probiotic bacteria are natural inhabitants of the intestinal flora and the vast majority of the strains and species that are examined in research for their probiotic properties are isolated from healthy humans although there are some that originate from fermented food.The increasing interest for replacement therapy has, however, opened a market for other consumer products such as lozenges, sucking tablets and chewing gums.

Probiotics are provided into the food items in one of four basic ways:

(i) as a culture concentrate added to beverages (e.g. fruit juice);

(ii) inoculated into prebiotic fibres which promote the growth of probiotic bacteria;

(iii) inoculated into milk and milkbased foods (e.g. milk drinks, yoghurt, cheese, kefifir, biodrinks); and

(iii) as lyophilized, dried cells packaged as dietary supplements (tablets, chewing gums, straws).

The archetypical probiotic food is yoghurt and daily consumption of dairy products seems to be the most natural way to ingest probiotic bacteria . Another advantage is that milk products contain basic nutrients for the growing child; they are also considered safe for the teeth with possible beneficial effects on the salivary microbial composition and inhibition of caries development, due to their natural content of casein, calcium, and phosphorous [113].

COLONIZATION AND SAFETY OF PROBIOTICS IN THE ORAL CAVITY

Some probiotic Lactobacillus and Streptococcus strains seem able to colonize the oral cavity of some people during the time that products containing them are in active use. However, both in vitro and in vivo evidence indicate that the differences between various probiotic strains, products, and also host individuals are obvious. L. rhamnosus GG and two different L. reuteri strains have been reported to colonize the oral cavity of 48–100% of volunteers consuming products containing them.In addition, S. salivarius K12, used for treating oral malodor, temporarily colonizes the oral cavity for a short time after use.

Some probiotic Lactobacillus and Streptococcus strains seem able to colonize the oral cavity of some people during the time that products containing them are in active use. However, both in vitro and in vivo evidence indicate that the differences between various probiotic strains, products, and also host individuals are obvious. L. rhamnosus GG and two different L. reuteri strains have been reported to colonize the oral cavity of 48–100% of volunteers consuming products containing them. In addition, S. salivarius K12, used for treating oral malodor, temporarily colonizes the oral cavity for a short time after use. Furthermore, consumption of a mixture of seven different Lactobacillus strains increased the number of salivary Lactobacillus counts, although the identities of the strains in the saliva were not determined. It seems feasible that probiotic bacteria would colonize the oral cavity only when they were used in products in contact with the mouth.

Indeed, Maukonen et al did not detect any of the probiotic bacteria administered in capsules in saliva samples. Surprisingly, consumption of capsules containing a mixture of seven different Lac tobacillus strains increased the number of salivary Lactobacillus counts. L. reuteri ATCC 55730 (= L.reuteri SD2112) does not seem to influence the total number of salivary lactobacilli, but L. rhamnosus GG may increase it [112].

OBSERVED EFFECTS ON ORAL HEALTH

1. Caries and caries-associated microbes [112]:

Several studies suggest that consumption of products containing probiotic lactobacilli or bifidobacteria could reduce the number of mutans streptococci in saliva. The tendency toward a decreased number of mutans streptococci in the saliva seems to be independent of the product or strain used; however, such effect has not been observed in all studies. The discrepancies between results cannot be explained by only the use of different probiotic strains, as different results have also been obtained using the same strains. In most of these studies, the levels of salivary lactobacilli have also been measured. With three products, an increase in the number of salivary Lactobacillus has been observed. Unfortunately, with respect to dental caries, the study groups have mainly been relatively small, and the studies fairly short. Furthermore, it is important to realize that the salivary level of caries-associated microbes does not equate to dental caries. In fact, the microbiota of unstimulated whole saliva resembles that of the tongue more than of dental plaque. Thus, no conclusive statement about the effects of probiotic bacteria on dental caries can be made.

2. Dental caries

Dental caries is one of the most prevalent chronic diseases of people worldwide and individuals are susceptible to this disease throughout their lifetime. Dental caries is a disease where the acids produced by bacterial metabolism of fermentable sugars causes damage to the hard tooth structure. Such damage is characterized by demineralization of the tooth enamel and dentin and leads to the formation of cavities on the surface of the tooth. Streptococcus mutans and Lactobacilli spp. are the most common bacteria involved in caries development. S. mutans has acidogenic properties and rapid metabolism of sucrose, fructose and glucose which generate low pH inducing cariogenic bacteria to establish in oral biofilm [114].

It should also be noted that as most probiotics are indairy forms containing high calcium, possibly reducing demineralization of teeth. Probiotics should adhere to dental tissues to establish a cariostatic effect and thus should be a part of the bio-film to fight the cariogenic bacteria [103].

To have a beneficial effect in controlling or preventing dental caries, a probiotic must adhere to dental surfaces and integrate into the dental plaque. It must also compete with and antagonize the cariogenic bacteria and thus inhibit their proliferation. Moreover, metabolism of dietary carbohydrates by the probiotic should result in no or low acid production [114].

Lactobacillus rhamnosus

Ahola and collaborators aimed to assess if short-term consumption of cheese containing L. rahmonosus GG (LGG) and L. rhamnosus LC 705 would reduce Streptococcus mutans levels. During the interventional period, the levels of S. mutans decreased in eight subjects (21%) of probiotic group and in seven (19%) of control group.Nase and collaborators turned down caries risk in school children through the use of a probiotic milk. The levels of S. mutans decreased in the test group and it was discovered that the caries risk in a subgroup of children, aging 3-4 years, was significantly reduced [114].

Lactobacillus reuteri

Several studies showed that L. reuteri has inhibitory properties towards S. mutans. These studies used different vehicles such as chewing gum, lozenge, straw, tablet and yogurt. It was demonstrated that different vehicles similarly exert inhibitory effects on the levels of S. mutans.

Caglar and collaborators tested a probiotic lozenge on 20 young healthy women this vehicle succeeded in reducing S. mutans count.Nikawa and collaborators evaluated the inhibitory effect of L reuteri against S. mutans, with special attention to the effect of a commercial yogurt containing L. reuteri on the oral carriage of S. mutans. The results obtained showed an antibacterial and inhibitory effect of the product against S. mutans in vitro and the reduction of the oral carriage of S. mutans in forty healthy and young subjects [114].

Bifidobacterium

Caglar and collaborators tested the effect of an ice cream containing Bifidobacterium lactis Bb-12 on the number of salivary mutans streptococci and lactobacilli. This protocol reduced the S. mutans counts but did not modify the lactobacilli ones.Cildir and collaborators tested the inhibitory effect of Bifidobacterium animalis subsp. lactis DN-173010 against S. mutans in patients with fixed orthodontic appliances. At the end of the study the test group showed a significant reduction of S. mutant counts compared to the controls, while the level of Bifidobacteria was unchanged [114].

3. Plaque [115]:

Dental plaque has been recognized as the single most important factor contributing to the etiology of dental caries. It is a cohort of micro-organisms involved in a wide range of physical, metabolic and molecular interactions. The plaque provides the pathogenic microorganisms with a favorable niche for growth and simultaneous protection from antimicrobial agents and host defenses. If not cleaned regularly, plaque can cause damage by buildup of tartar leading to gum problems, tooth decay and even tooth loss.

Probiotics reduce plaque induction by neutralizing free electrons, modulating systemic immune system and also by regulating mucosal permeability. Strains of Streptococcus thermophilus and Lactococcus lactis strains were shown to adhere to saliva coated hydroxyapatite beads in an in-vitro study. L. lactis NCC2211 successfully incorporates itself into a biofilm, thus mimicking the dental plaque, and modulates the growth of the cariogenic Streptococcus sobrinus OMZ176.

4. Periodontal Disease

Periodontal disease has been described as "a heterogeneous group of pathoses characterized by a predominance of specific infectious agents in the face of inadequate local host defenses" [37] where the balance between protective and destructive immune responses is a key determinant of disease progression. Periodontal disease can be classified into two types: gingivitis (inflammation of the gingiva) and periodontitis (progressive disease that affects all supporting tissues of the teeth).

The accumulation of bacteria within the biofilm, facilitated by poor oral hygiene, predisposes to allogenic shifts in the microbial community, leading to the onset of periodontal inflammation. Gram-negative anaerobic microorganisms are considered to be pathogenic to the dental-supporting tissues. They cause intense inflammation which triggers destruction of the soft connective tissue and the underlying alveolar bone and ligament supporting the teeth. The main pathogenic agents associated with periodontitis are P. gingivalis, Treponema denticola, Tannerella forsythia and Aggregatibacter actinomycetemcomitans.

In vitro, A. actinomycetemcomitans and P. gingivalis are pathogens associated with elevate production of metallo proteases-2 (MMP-2) that could be responsible for tissue destruction and disin tegration of extracellular matrix in periodontal diseases [114].

The first studies of the use of probiotics for enhancing oral health were for the treatment of periodontal inflammation. Patients with various periodontal diseases, gingivitis, periodontitis, and pregnancy gingivitis, were locally treated with a culture supernatant of a L. acidophilus strain. Significant recovery was reported for almost every patient.

The probiotic strains used in these studies include L. reuteri strains, L. brevis (CD2), L. casei Shirota, L. salivarius WB21, and Bacillus subtilis. L. reuteri and L. brevis have improved gingival health, as measured by decreased gum bleeding.The use of probiotic chewing gum containing L. reuteri ATCC 55730 and ATCC PTA 5289 also decreased levels of pro-inflammatory cytokines in GCF, and the use of L. brevis decreased MMP (collagenase) activity and other inflammatory markers in saliva. With L. casei Shirota and Bacillus subtilis no difference in test and control groups in gingival bleeding or measured plaque index was observed, but the use of L. casei Shirota decreased PMN elastase and MMP-3 activities in GCF, and gingival inflammation was lower in the group consuming the probiotic product, as measured by MPO activity after a four-day period of experimental gingivitis. B. subtilis seemed to reduce the number of periodontal pathogens.Use of tablets containing L. salivarius WB21 has been shown to decrease gingival pocket depth, particularly in high-risk groups such as smokers, and also affect the number of periodontopathogens in plaque.Again, although encouraging results have been observed, most studies have been fairly short. Furthermore, in some studies the observed differences were quite small, though statistically significant [112].

Gudrianov and collaborators have shown that periodontal inflammation is reduced by the ingestion of tables containing probiotic Bifidumbacterin and Acilact. Lactobacillus brevis was studied in a group of patients with chronic periodontitis demonstrating that 4 days of sucking lozenges improved plaque and gingival index and bleeding on probing for all patients. This seems due to the effect of L. brevis on the prevention of production of nitric oxide (NO) which posi tively regulates salivary levels of prostaglandin E2 (PGE2) and matrix MMPs [114].

According to Koll-Klais et al, high levels of Lactobacillus in microbiota caused an 82% and 65% inhibition in Porphyromonas gingivalis and Prevotella intermedia growth, respectively. In a study published in 2005, the prevalence of lactobacilli, particularly Lactobacillus gasseri and Lactobacillus fermentum, in the oral cavity was greater among healthy participants than among patients with chronic periodontitis[103].

The currently available data indicate an effect of probiotics on periodontal pathogens and clinical periodontal parameters.

5. Nitrate-Reducing Bacteria as Probiotic Agents [116]:

Nitric oxide (NO) is a labile and highly reactive gas which is known to be generated endogenously through the activity of NO synthases from mammalian cells and contributes to host defence against a number of pathogenic microorganisms. Nitrate absorbed from ingested dietary sources, especially green vegetables, is actively concentrated by the salivary glands so that concentrations in the saliva are approximately 10 times those found in plasma. Nitrate is then rapidly converted to nitrite in the mouth by bacteria, through the activity of nitrate reductase enzymes. It has been shown that the bacteria responsible for nitrate reduction reside within the crypts of the tongue, where they are maintained in an anaerobic environment and reduce nitrate to nitrite during respiration.High concentrations of nitrite formed in saliva will, when acidified in the stomach, produce nitrous acid and NO in sufficient concentrations to kill Escherichia coli and other enteric pathogens. Additionally salivary nitrite will encounter the acid environment around the teeth provided by acidogenic bacteria such as Lactobacillus spp. and Streptococcus mutans.

A relationship between dental caries and levels of nitrate and microbial nitrate reductase activity in the saliva of children has been established. Compared with control subjects, a eduction in caries experience was found in patients with high salivary nitrate and high nitrate-reducing ability. In man, the new-born infant is at first edentulous and has a microbial flora characteristic of this condition. Studies have shown that the frequency of isolation of NRB significantly increases after the teeth begin to erupt at about the age of 6 months. Thus, probiotic therapy could be accomplished by the introduction of NRB into neonates, which have yet to acquire these bacteria or adults after the use of broad-spectrum antibiotics to firstly reduce tongue populations of bacteria.

It is well established that salivary glands may respond to periodontitis through the enhancement of the protective effects of saliva. An increase in nitrate secretion and subsequent increase in salivary nitrite through the activity of NRB has been found to be higher in subjects with periodontitis and thus may contribute to this protection in response to the inflammatory process. NO levels in saliva and gingival crevicular fluid have been found to be higher in patients with aggressive periodontitis as compared to gingivitis. This could arise both through an increase in salivary nitrate and subsequent microbial reduction and also through the activity of host NO synthases where the upregulation of enzyme activity in response to periodontal bacteria has been shown.

Therefore the use of probiotics to enhance oral NO production through both nitrate reduction and upregulation of synthase activity may be beneficial in the control of bacteria associated with dental caries and periodontitis.

6. Candida infection:

Probiotics are used to control Candida infection in elderly patient since elderly are more prone to candida infection provoked by chronic diseases, medications, poor oral hygiene, reduced salivary flow and impaired immune response. Bacteria like Lactococcus lactis, Lactobacillus helveticus, Lactobacillus rhamnosus GG (ATCC53103), Lactobacillus rhamnosus LC705 when used in one of the study, showed significant reduction of candida infection[103].

When a test group of elderly people consumed cheese containing L. rhamnosus strains GG and LC705 and Propionibacterium freudenreichii ssp. shermanii JS for 16 weeks, the number of high oral yeast counts decreased, but no changes were observed in mucosal lesions. In a shorter study with younger subjects, no significant difference was observed between effects of probiotic and those of control cheese on salivary Candida counts [112].

7. Hyposalivation and xerostomia

Evidence suggests that probiotics can also reduce the risk of hypo-salivation and feeling of dry mouth[103].

8. Probiotics and halitosis

Halitosis is a general term used to define an unpleasant odor emanating from the breath. In vast majority of the cases, halitosis is caused by oral conditions and is known as oral malodour. Oral malodour is a common condition which affects a large proportion of the human adult population, although it can occur in people of all ages. It is generally not considered to be a medical concern, but it can significantly impact normal social interactions. Halitosis is the result of the release of malodouros substances into the breath [15].

The most common malodouros substances are

(i) by-products of the metabolism of certain oral bacteria species, including volatile sulphur compounds (VSC; hydrogen sulphide, methyl mercaptan and dimethyl sulphide).

(ii) short-chain fatty acids (butyric acid, valeric acid, propionic acid), phenyl compounds (indole, skatole, pyridiene), and diamines (putrescine, cadaverine).

(iii) The oral organisms are proteolytic, anaerobe Gram negative bacteria, mainly located on the tongue dorsum and/or residing in periodontal pockets. These bacteria include Porphyromonas gingivalis, Prevotella intermedia, Fusobacterium nucleatum, Micromonas micros, Campylobacter rectus, Eikenella corrodens and Treponema denticola, as well as Tannerella forsythia and various species of Bacteroides, Desulfovibrio and Eubacterium [114].

Probiotics are marketed for the treatment of both mouth- and gut-associated halitosis. Despite that, only a few clinical studies have found different probiotic strains or products to be efficacious. The studied strains include E. coliNisle 1917, S. salivarius K12, three Weissella confusa isolates, and a lactic acid–forming bacterial mixture, not specified by the authors of that work [112].

Regular use of probiotics can help to control halitosis. After taking Weissella cibaria, reduced levels of volatile sulfide components produced by Fusobacterium nucleatum were observed by Kang et al. The effect could be due to hydrogen peroxide production by Weissella cibaria, causing Fusobacterium nucleatum inhibition[103].

The studies currently available on the effects of oral administration of probiotics on oral malodour did not provide definitive results, as all of them are pilot/preliminary investigations, with some limitations such as small number of participants and short intervention period. The results obtained, however, are encouraging and therefore highlight the need to design and conduct further large scale randomized clinical trial [114].

Clinical trails should be directed to assess the method of probiotic administration in oral cavity and dosages for different therapeutic uses. Research should be directed towards the action of probiotics on oral cavity and also on its pathological conditions.

PROBLEMS AND RECOMMENDATIONS IN ORAL PROBIOTIC RESEARCH [110]:

Problem	Recommendation/ comment
Complex microbiology of the oral cavity	Systematic screening for potential resident probiotic strains. Interactions between microorganisms of the mouth are poorly understood
Different microbial attachment sites	Investigating microbial (probiotic) attachment separately on the teeth, and on keratinized and non-keratinized epithelium. Probably different probiotics are needed for therapy in dental and oral mucosal diseases
Saliva	Salivary defense mechanisms, both specific and nonspecific, should be investigated in relation to potential probiotics. Data from gastrointestinal studies are not directly applicable in saliva parameters
Safety	Strains that readily ferment dietary carbohydrates and decrease pH in the mouth are not suitable probiotics for oral health purposes. In addition, general safety aspects such as those related to potential invasiveness and antibiotic resistance genes must be screened
Means of administration and dosage	Slow-release approach should be investigated. It appears that probiotic therapy in order to be effective needs to be continuously administered. Optimal dosages of probiotics in oral health indications need to be assessed
Trials	Randomized controlled trails are needed with patients materials based on proper power calculations. Probiotic intervention should be tested in the clinical setting using potential strains for specific oral health purposes
Genetically modified microorganisms	Whether or not potentially probiotic microbial strains can or should be genetically modified in order to strengthen their beneficial potential or characteristics needs to be investigated. In the first hand, this calls for extensive studies on the mechanisms of probiotic action

Table 9: Problems And Recommendations In Oral Probiotic Research

FUTURE ASPECTS

Novel probiotic solutions, targeting oral health, constitute a new class of products that are a great leap beyond the conventional over the counter solutions. With the changing lifestyle and feeding habits, globally, it is anticipated that rise in oral diseases will be proportional to other lifestyle diseases. Identification of strains from indigenous fermented products such as kefir, curd, etc. followed by rigorous preclinical and clinical trials can help generate novel probiotic with desired effects. These natural strains can reduce our dependency on chemical based interventions for daily upkeep of oral health and prevention of diseases. Similarly, for serious oral diseases genetically modified microbes may open up a whole new dimension to the concept of probiotics in the near future. The strain can be modified to encompass biofilm formation, bacteriocin production etc. and simultaneously endure the feeding habits of the host. Alternatively, the said strains could be used to enhance the properties of a natural oral microbiota. Host oral microbiota characterization can also be a possibility in the near future to understand the underlying conditions. This can help deciding the treatment options or therapy to shift the balance towards the beneficial microbiota.

However, all the products effective in oral health care are required to be administered daily, so a possible way of administration could be to incorporate probiotics in toothpaste, mouthwash, chewing gums, sugar-less candy for kids etc. Some of these products are already available over-the-counter in western countries and are fast gaining popularity in others [115].

Oral lactic acid bacteria and bifidobacteria have been isolated and characterized for various oral health purposes, including caries, periodontal diseases, and halitosis. In addition, dairy strains have been studied with the aim of characterizing potential new oral probiotics; thus, the new probiotic products targeted for oral health purposes do not necessarily comprise the same species as products now in market. Furthermore, the species might not necessarily belong only to genera Lactobacillus or Bifidobacteium. Indeed, S. salivarius K12 is used to treat oral malodor,55 and preliminary results have been published on the safety and efficacy of a probiotic mouthwash containing three different oral streptococci for reducing the number of bacteria associated with dental caries and periodontitis.

Genetically modified microbes bring a new dimension to the concept of probiotics. One approach is to reduce the harmful properties of pathogenic strains naturally colonizing the oral cavity. The modified strain could then be used to replace the original pathogen. One ambitious and promising example is the generation of an S. mutans strain with a complete deletion of the open reading frame of lactate hydrogenase and thus significantly reduced cariogenicity. Another option could be to enhance the properties of a potentially beneficial strain. One example is the construction of an L. paracasei strain with a functional scFV (single-chain variable fragment) antibody binding to the surface of Porphyromonas gingivalis [112].

CONCLUSION

Oral health has a direct impact on an individual's well-being and quality of life. Oral diseases can limit the individual's capacity of eating, speaking and smiling thereby greatly damaging personal and social life [115]. Probiotics represent a new area of research in oral healthcare. The examination of the close relationships between diet and oral health could potentially be regulated with a variety of different products as: conventional foods (for consumption by general population), dietary supplements (the products are meant to be used as oral supplements to the diet, and are not to be represented as meals), medical foods (foods used under medical supervision for patients needing special dietary support for medical condition.), drugs (meant to cure, treat, mitigate, prevent, diagnose or cure disease) and feed additives [114].

Bacteriotherapy in the form of probiotics seems to be a natural way to maintain health and protect oral tissues from disease, and data suggest that the potential benefits increase with an early childhood start. The research is still in its infancy but a daily intake of probiotic lactobacilli with an inhibitory effect on other bacteria is currently most promising. Milk, milk drinks, or yoghurt containing one or more probiotic strains could be a treatment option in the long-term prevention of childhood caries [113].

Probiotic bacterium in the mouth is not necessarily an oral probiotic. Furthermore, it is quite possible that the same species are not optimal for all oral health purposes; e.g., different properties might be desired in respect to dental and gingival health.some of the probiotic bacteria used in various probiotic products may colonize the oral cavity during the time they are in use; thus, the effects of probiotic bacteria in the oral cavity are important to understand. Probiotic bacteria seem to affect both oral microbiota and immune responses. On the other hand, the extent to which bacteria in food or in food ingredients can influence relatively stable oral microbiota is difficult to predict [112].

Evidence of beneficial effects of probiotics on oral health is accumulating. In general, the growing population awareness and demand for healthy living inevitably leads to broader availability of health-promoting foods in the market. In this field probiotics have become fashionable among the public and are marketed as one of the key elements in well-balanced general health. As discussed here, most oral health effects of probiotics have been observed after administration of strains which are not natural members of oral microbiota. Possibly a more attractive and reliable probiotic might be found among species which are natural members in the host microbiome. Screening of such probiotic candidates in human oral bacterial populations is ongoing with some evidence already available. Further, multi-center clinical trials with enough statistical power, and the use of high-throughput analytical tools, are needed for true evidence before the role of probiotics on oral health can be established and their use justified. Currently the evidence yet remains weak [105].

REFERENCES

1. Bagchi T. Traditional food & modern lifestyle: impact of probiotics. Indian J Med Res. 2014;140(3):333e5.

2. M. M. Toma and J. Pokrotnieks. Probiotics as functional food: microbiological and medical aspects. Acta Universitatis. 2006; 710: 117–129.

3. S. J. Salminen, M. Gueimonde, and E. Isolauri. Probiotics that modify disease risk. Journal of Nutrition. 2005;135 (5):1294–1298.

4. Soccol CR, Vandenberghe LPS, Spier MR, Medeiros ABP, Yamaguishi CT, Lindrier JD et al. The Potential of Probiotics, Food Technol. Biotechnol. 2010; 48 (4):413–434.

5. Tannock GW. Normal microflora. An Introduction to Microbes Inhabiting the Human Body, London: Chapman & Hall, 1995.

6. Zoetendal EG, Akkermans ADL, Akkermans-van Vliet WM et al. The host genotype affects the bacterial community in the human gastrointestinal tract. Microbial Ecology in Health and Disease. 2001; 13: 129–134.

7. Isolauri E. Probiotics. Best Practice & Research Clinical Gastroenterology. 2004; 18(2) : 299-313.

8. Larsen B & Monif GRG. Understanding the bacterial flora of the female genital tract. Clinical Infectious Diseases.2001; 32: e69–e77.

9. Benno Y & Mitsuoka T. Development of intestinal microflora in humans and animals. Bifidobacteria and Microflora.1986; 5: 13–25.

10. Gronlund MM, Lehtonen OP, Eerola E & Kero P. Fecal microflora in healthy infants born by different methods of delivery: permanent changes in intestinal flora after Cesarean delivery. Journal of Pediatric Gastroenterology and Nutrition. 1999; 28: 19–25.

11. Harmsen HJM, Wildeboer-Veloo ACM, Raangs GC et al. Analysis of intestinal flora development in breast-fed and formula-fed infants by using molecular identifification and detection methods. Journal of Pediatric Gastroenterology and Nutrition. 2000; 30: 61–67.

12. Favier CF, Vaughan EE, de Vos WM & Akkermans ADL. Molecular monitoring of succession of bacterial communities in human neonates. Applied and Environmental Microbiology.2002; 68: 219–226.

13. Vaughan E, de Vries M, Zoetendal E et al. The intestinal LABs. Anthonie van Leeuwenhoek. 2002; 82: 341–352.

14. Tannock GW. Analysis of the intestinal microflflora: a renaissance. Anthonie van Leeuwenhoek.1999; 76: 265–278.

15. Zoetendal EG, Akkermans AD & de Vos WM. Temperature gradient gel electrophoresis analysis of 16S rRNA from human faecal samples reveals stable and host-specific communities of active bacteria. Applied and Environmental Microbiology.1998; 64: 3854–3859.

16. Mitsuoka T. Bififidobacteria and their role in human health. Journal of Industrial Microbiolology. 1990; 6: 263–267.

17. Hopkins MJ & Macfarlane GT. Changes in predominanat bacterial populations in human faeces with age and with Clostridium difficile infection. Journal of Medical Microbiology.2002; 51: 448–454.

18. Andrieux C, Membre´ JM, Cayuela C & Antoine JM. Metabolic characteristics of the faecal microflora in humans from three age groups. Scandinavian Journal of Gastroenterology.2002; 37: 792–798.

19. Patel RM, Denning PW. Therapeutic use of prebiotics, probiotics, and postbiotics to prevent necrotizing enterocolitis: what is the current evidence?. Clin Perinatol.2013;40:11e25.

20. Islam SU. Clinical uses of probiotics. Medicine (Baltimore) 2016;95:1-5.

21. Ooi MF, Mazlan N, Foo HL, Loh TC, Mohamad R, Rahim RA, et al. Effects of carbon and nitrogen sources on bacteriocininhibitory activity of postbiotic metabolites produced by Lactobacillus plantarum I-UL4. Malays J Microbiol. 2015;11:176-184.

22. Giorgetti GM, Brandimarte G, Fabiocchi F, Ricci S, Flamini P, Sandri G, et al. Interactions between innate immunity, microbiota, and probiotics. J Immunol Res 2015;501361:7.

23. G. R. Gibson and M. B. Roberfroid, "Dietary modulation of the human colonic microbiota: introducing the concept of prebiotics," Journal of Nutrition. 1995; 125(6):1401–1412.

24. Cicenia A, Scirocco A, Carabotti M, Pallotta L, Marignani M, Severi C. Postbiotic activities of lactobacilli-derived factors. J Clin Gastroenterol.2014;48:S18e22.

25. Pokusaeva K, Fitzgerald GF, van Sinderen D.Carbohydrate metabolism in Bifidobacteria. Gen Nutr. 6(3):285–306.

26. Rastall RA, Gibson GR. Recent developments in prebiotics to selectively impact beneficial microbes and promote intestinal health. Curr Opinion Biotechnol. 2015;32:42e6.

27. Thomas LV. Probiotics-the journey continues. Int J Dairy Tech. 2016;69:1e12.

28. Hutkins RW, Krumbeck JA, Bindels LB, Cani PD, Fahey G, Goh YJ, et al. Prebiotics: why defifinitions matter. Curr Opin Biotechnol. 2016;37:1e13.

29. Tanaka R, Takayama H, Morotomi M, Kuroshima T, Ueyama S, Matsumoto K, et al. Effects of administration of TOS and Bififidobacterium breve 4006 on the human fecal flora. Bififidobact Microflora. 1983;2:17e24.

30. Pena AS. Intestinal flora, probiotics, prebiotics, synbiotics and novel foods. Rev Esp Enferm Dig. 2007;99:653e8.

31. Swennen K, Courtin CM, Delcour JA. Non-digestible oligosaccharides with prebiotic properties. Crit Rev Food Sci Nutr. 2006; 46(6): 459–471.

32. Villamiel M, Montilla A, Olano A, Corzo N. Production and bioactivity of oligosaccharides derived from lactose. In: Moreno FJ, Sanz ML, editors. Food oligosaccharides: production, analysis and bioactivity. Wiley Blackwell; 2014. p. 137e67.

33. Trollope KM, van Wyk N, Kotjomela MA, Volschenk H. Sequence and structure-based prediction of fructosyltransferase activity for functional sub classifification of fungal GH32 enzymes. FEBS J. 2015;282:4782e96.

34. Collins S, Reid G. Distant site effects of ingested prebiotics. Nutrients. 2016;8:523.

35. Zhou Y, Kruger C, Ravi GS, Kumar DPS, Vijayasarathi SK, Lavingia M, et al. Safety evaluation of galactooligosaccharides: sub chronic oral toxicity study in Sprague-Dawley rats. Toxicol Res Appl.2017;1:1e12.

36. Pretorius R, Prescott SL, Palmer DJ. Taking a prebiotic approach to early immunomodulation for allergy prevention. Expert Rev Clin Immunol.2018;14(1):43e51.

37. Kerry, Rout & Patra, Jayanta Kumar & Gouda, Sushanto & Park, Yooheon & Shin, Hanseung & Das,. (2018). Benefaction of probiotics for human health: A review. Journal of Food and Drug Analysis. 26. 10.1016/j.jfda.2018.01.002.

38. DeVrese M, Schrezenmeir J. (2008) Probiotics, prebiotics, and synbiotics. in food biotechnology. Springer Berlin Heidelberg (pp. 1–66)

39. Gibson GR, Roberfroid MB. Dietary modulation of the human colonic microbiota: introducing the concept of prebiotics. J Nutr. 1995;125:1401e12.

40. Romeo J, Nova E, Wärnberg J, Gómez-Martínez S, DíazLigia LE, Marcos A. Immunomodulatory effect of fibres, probiotics and synbiotics in different life-stages.Nutr Hosp. 2010; 25(3):341–9

41. Zhang MM, Cheng JQ, Lu YR, Yi ZH, Yang P, Wu XT. Use of pre-, pro-and synbiotics in patients with acute pancreatitis: a metaanalysis. World J Gastroenterol. 2010; 16(31):3970.

42. R. Fuller. Probiotics in man and animals. Journal of Applied Bacteriology. 1989; 66(5) :365–378.

43. D.M. Lilly, R.H. Stillwell. Probiotics: Growth-promoting factors produced by microorganisms. Science. 1965; 47 : 747–748.

44. J. Fioramonti, V. Theodorou, L. Bueno. Probiotics: What are they? What are their effects on gut physiology?. Best Pract. Res. Clin. Gastroenterol. 2003; 17 : 711–724.

45. S. Salminen, A. von Wright, L. Morelli, P. Marteau, D. Brassart, W.M. de Vos, R. Fondén, M. Saxelin, K. Collins, G. Mogensen, S.E. Birkeland, T. Mattila-Sandholm. Demonstration of safety of probiotics – A review. Int. J. Food Microbiol. 1998; 44 : 93–106.

46. P.R. Marteau, M. de Vrese, C.J. Cellier, J. Schrezenmeir. Protection from gastrointestinal diseases with the use of probiotics. Am. J. Clin. Nutr. 2001; 73: 430–436.

47. W.P. Charteris, P.M. Kelly, L. Morelli, J.K. Collins. Selective detection,enumeration and identification of potentially probiotic Lactobacillus and Bifidobacterium species in mixed bacterial populations. Int. J. Food Microbiol. 1997; 35: 1–27.

48. FAO/WHO, Report on Joint FAO/WHO Expert Consultation on Evaluation of Health and Nutritional Properties of Probiotics in Food Including Powder Milk with Live Lactic Acid Bacteria, 2001.

49. A.Hosono. Fermented Milk in the Orient. In: Functions of Fermented Milk: Challenges for the Health Sciences, Y. Nagasawa, A. Hosono (Eds.), Elsevier Applied Science, London, UK (1992) pp. 61–78.

50. C. Shortt, The probiotic century: Historical and current perspectives, Trends Food Sci. Technol.1999; 10: 411–417.

51. I.I. Metchnikoff, P. Chalmers Mitchel. Nature of Man or Studies in Optimistic Philosophy, Kessinger Publishing, Whitefish, MT, USA (1910).

52. I.I. Metchnikoff: The Prolongation of Life: Optimistic Studies, Springer Publishing Company, NewYork, NY, USA (2004).

53. M. Del Piano, L. Morelli, G.P. Strozzi, S. Allesina, M. Barba, F. Deidda et al. Probiotics: From research to consumer. Dig. Liv. Dis.2006, 38 (2): 248–255.

54. W.L. Kulp, L.F. Rettger. Comparative study of Lactobacillus acidophilus and Lactobacillus bulgaricus. J. Bacteriol. 1924; 9: 357–395.

55. H.Cheplin, L. Rettger. The therapeutic application of Lactobacillus acidophilus. Abs. Bact. 1922; 6 :24.

56. Lactobacillus casei strain Shirota, Yakult Honsha Co. Ltd, Yakult Central Institute for Microbiological Research, Tokyo, Japan (1998).

57. DeVrese M, Schrezenmeir J. (2008) Probiotics, prebiotics, and synbiotics. in food biotechnology (pp. 1–66). Springer Berlin Heidelberg

58. Harmsen HJ, Wildeboer-Veloo AC, Raangs GC, Wagendorp AA, Klijn N, Bindels JG, *et al*. Analysis of intestinal flora development in breast –fed and formula –fed infants by using molecular identification and detection methods. J Pediatr Gastroenterol Nutr. 2000;30:61-7.

59. Salminen S, Von Wright A, Morelli L, Marteau P, Brassart D, De Vos WM, et al. Demonstration of safety of probiotics-a review.Int J Food Microbiol.1998; 44: 93-106

60. Kechagia M, Basoulis D, Konstantopoulou S, Dimitriadi D, Gyftopoulou K, Skarmoutsou N, Fakiri EM. Health Benefits of Probiotics: A Review. ISRN Nutrition. 2013; 1-7.

61. Isolauri E, Saliminen S, Ouwehand AC. Probiotics: An overview of beneficial effects. Antonie van Leeuwenhoek. 2002; 82: 279-289

62. Natural Medicines Comprehensive Database. *Lactobacillus* monograph.www.naturaldatabase.com (accessed 2022 Mar 23).

63. Natural Medicines Comprehensive Database. Bifidobacteria monograph. www. naturaldatabase.com (accessed 2022 Mar 23).

64. Natural Medicines Comprehensive Database. *Saccharomyces boulardii* monograph. www.naturaldatabase.com (accessed 2022 April 9).

65. Gupta V, Garg R. Probiotics. Indian Journal of Medical Microbiology. 2009; 27(3): 202-9.

66. Williams NT. Probiotics. Am J Health-Syst Pharm. 2010; 67: 449-458.

67. Aureli P, Capurso L , Castellazzi AM, Clerici M, Giovannini M, Morelli L et al.. Probiotics and health: An evidence-based review. Pharmacological Research. 2011; 63:366–376.

68. Food and Agriculture Organization/World Health Organization (FAO/WHO), Guidelines for the evaluation of probiotics in food, Report of a Joint FAO/WHO Working Group on Drafting Guidelines

for the Evaluation of Probiotics in Food, London, Ontario, Canada (2002) (http://ftp.fao.org/es/esn/food/wgreport2.pdf).

69. N.P. Shah. Functional cultures and health benefits. Int. Dairy J. 2007; 17: 1262–1277.

70. J. Chow. Probiotics and prebiotics: A brief overview. J. Ren. Nutr. 2002; 12: 76–86.

71. Kerry RG, Patra JK, Gouda S, Park Y, Shin HS, Das G. Benefaction of probiotics for human health: A review. Journal of food and drug analysis. 2018; 26(3):927-939

72. B. Sgorbati, B. Biavati, D. Palenzona. The Genus Bifidobacterium. In: The Lactic Acid Bacteria, Vol. 2, B.J.B. Wood, W.H. Holzapfel (Eds.), Chapman and Hall, London, UK (1995) pp. 279–306.

73. A.M.P. Gomes, F.X. Malcata. Bifidobacterium spp. and Lactobacillus acidophilus: Biological, biochemical, technological and therapeutical properties relevant for use as probiotics. Trends Food Sci. Technol. 1999; 10: 139–157.

74. S.M. Finegold, V.L. Sutter, G.E. Mathisen. Normal Indigenous Intestinal Flora. In: Human Intestinal Microflora in Health and Disease, D.J. Hentges (Ed.), Academic Press, New York, NY, USA (1983) pp. 3–31.

75. W.P. Hammes, R.F. Vogel: The Genus Lactobacillus. In: The Lactic Acid Bacteria, Vol. 2, B.J.B. Wood, W.H. Holzapfel (Eds.), Chapman and Hall, London, UK (1995) pp. 19–54.

76. S. Salminen, E. Isolauri, E. Salminen. Clinical uses of probiotics for stabilizing the gut mucosal barrier: Successful strains and future challenges. Antonie van Leeuwenhoek. 1996; 70: 347–358.

77. Cutting SM. Bacillus probiotics. Food Microbiol. 2011 Apr;28(2):214-20

78. T.M. Barbosa, C.R. Serra, R.M. La Ragione, M.J. Woodward, A.O. Henriques. Screening for Bacillus isolates in the broiler gastrointestinal tract, Appl. Environ. Microbiol.2005; 71: 968–978.

79. F. Coppi, M. Ruoppolo, A. Mandressi, C. Bellorofonte, G. Gonnella, A. Trinchieri. Results of treatment with Bacillus subtilis spores (Enterogermina) after antibiotic therapy in 95 patients with infection calculosis. Chemioterapia.1985; 4 :467–470.

80. Mandel DR, Eichas K, Holmes J. Bacillus coagulans: a viable adjunct therapy for relieving symptoms of rheumatoid arthritis according to a randomized, controlled trial. BMC Complement Altern Med. 2010 Jan 12;10:1

81. T. Hosoi, K. Kiuchi: Production and Probiotic Effects of Natto. In: Bacterial Spore Formers: Probiotics and Emerging Applications, E. Ricca, A.O. Henriques, S.M. Cutting (Eds.), Horizon Bioscience, Wymondham, UK (2004) pp. 143–154.

82. H. Sumi, C. Yatagai, H. Wada, E. Yoshida, M. Maruyama. Effect of Bacillus natto-fermented product (BIOZYME) on blood alcohol, aldehyde concentrations after whisky drinking in human volunteers, and acute toxicity of acetaldehyde in mice. Arukoru Kenkyuto Yakubutsu Ison. 1995; 30: 69–79.

83. R. Fuller. Probiotics in human medicine. Gut. 1991; 32 : 439–442.

84. R.M. La Ragione, G. Casula, S.M. Cutting, S.M. Woodward. Bacillus subtilis spores competitively exclude Escherichia coli 070:K80 in poultry. Vet. Microbiol. 2001; 79: 133–142.

85. B. Vaseeharan, P. Ramasamy. Control of pathogenic Vibriospp. by Bacillus subtilis BT23, a possible probiotic treatment for black tiger shrimp Penaeus monodon. Lett. Appl. Microbiol. 2003; 36: 83–87.

86. S.M. Fox. Probiotics: Intestinal inoculants for production animals. Vet. Med. 1988; 83: 806–830.

87. O.B. Maia, R. Duarte, A.M. Silva, D.C. Cara, J.R. Nicoli. Evaluation of the components of a commercial probiotic in gnotobiotic mice experimentally challenged with Salmonella enterica subsp. enterica ser. Typhimurium. Vet. Microbiol. 2001; 79 :183–189.

88. The effect of a probiotic milk product on plasma cholesterol: A meta-analysis of short-term intervention studies, Eur. J. Clin. Nutr. 2000; 54: 856–860.

89. C. Wendt, B. Wiesenthal, E. Dietz, H. Rüden. Survival of vancomycin-resistant and vancomycin-susceptible enterococci on dry surfaces. J. Clin. Microbiol. 1998; 36: 3734– 3736.

90. M. Lara-Flores, M.A. Olvera-Novoa, B.E. Guzmán-Méndez, W. López-Madrid. Use of the bacteria Streptococcus faecium and Lactobacillus acidophilus, and the yeast Saccharomyces cerevisiae as growth promoters in Nile tilapia (Oreochromis niloticus). Aquaculture. 2003; 216: 193–201.

91. A. van der Aa Kühle, K. Skovgaard, L. Jespersen. In vitro screening of probiotic properties of Saccharomyces cerevisiae var. boulardii and food-borne Saccharomyces cerevisiae strains. Int. J. Food Microbiol. 2005; 101:29–39.

92. C. Lacroix, S. Yildirim, Fermentation technologies for the production of probiotics with high viability and functionality, Curr. Opin. Biotechnol.2007; 18: 176–183.

93. Pandey KR, Naik SR, Vakil BV. Probiotics, prebiotics and synbiotics- a review. J Food Sci Technol. 2015 Dec;52(12):7577-87.

94. Jain P and Sharma P. Probiotics and Their Efficacy in Improving Oral Health: A Review.Journal of Applied Pharmaceutical Science. 2012; 2 (11): 151-163.

95. S. Scheinbach, Probiotics: Functionality and commercial status, Biotechnol. Adv. 1998; 16: 581–608

96. A.Y. Tamime, M. Saarela, A. Korslund Søndergaard, V.V. Mistry, N.P. Shah. Production and Maintenance of Viability of Probiotic Micro-Organisms in Dairy Products. In: Probiotic Dairy Products, A.Y. Tamime (Ed.), Blackwell Publishing, Oxford, UK (2005) pp. 44–51.

97. A. Lourens-Hattingh, B.C. Viljoen, Yogurt as probiotic carrier food, Int. Dairy J. 2011; 11: 1–17.

98. S. Lye, C.Y. Kuan, J.A. Ewe, W.Y. Fung, M.T. Liong, The improvement of hypertension by probiotics: Effects on cholesterol, diabetes, Renin, and phytoestrogens, Int. J. Mol. Sci. 2009; 27: 3755–3775.

99. A.K. Goel, N. Dilbaghi, D.V. Kamboj, L. Singh, Probiotics: Microbial therapy for health modulation, Defence Sci. J. 2006; 56: 513–529.

100.Bäckhed, Addressing the gut microbiome and implications for obesity, Int. Dairy J. 2010; 20: 259–261.

101.P.D. Cani, A.M. Neyrinck, F. Fava, C. Knauf, R.G. Burcelin, K.M. Tuohy et al. Selective increases of bifidobacteria in gut microflora improve high-fat-diet-induced diabetes in mice through a mechanism associated with endotoxaemia. Diabetologia. 2007; 50: 2374–2383.

102.M. E. Falagas, G. I. Betsi, and S. Athanasiou. Probiotics for the treatment of women with bacterial vaginosis. Clinical Microbiology and Infection. 2007; 13(7): 657–664.